KUNDALINI AWAKENING

A Visual Journey In Meditation

Santosh Sachdeva

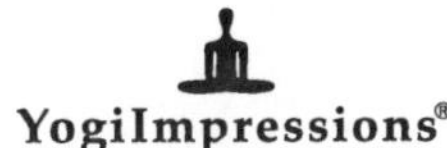
YogiImpressions®

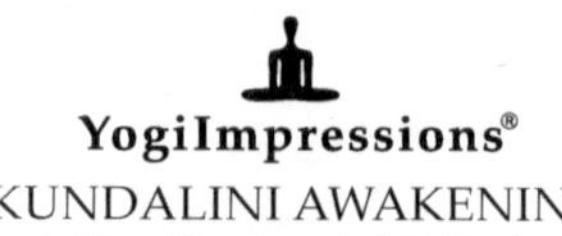

KUNDALINI AWAKENING
A Visual Journey In Meditation

First published in India in 2005 by
Yogi Impressions LLP
1711, Centre 1, World Trade Centre,
Cuffe Parade, Mumbai 400 005, India.
Website: www.yogiimpressions.com

First Edition, June 2005
Twelfth reprint: February 2024

ISBN 978-81-88479-68-9

Printed at: Thomson Press (I) Ltd.

CONTENTS

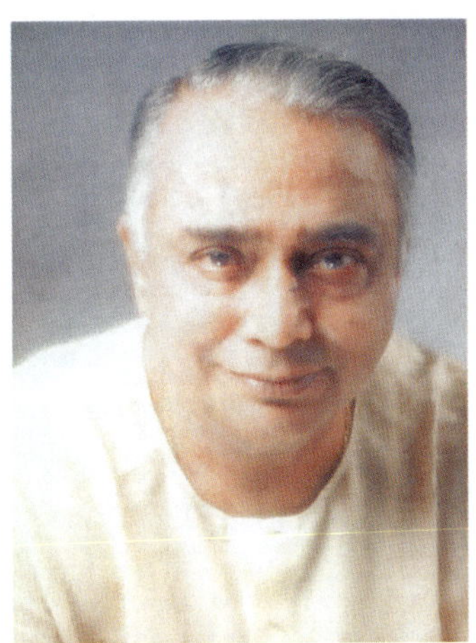

Justice M. L. Dudhat

Dedicated to Guruji,
the Yogis on our plane,
those from other realms,
and all Seekers.

ACKNOWLEDGEMENTS

I wish to express, with love and joy, my deepest gratitude to:

My *Guru,* Shri M. L. Dudhat, under whose guidance my spiritual growth took place.

Swami Ramanathan for his love, gentleness, and support.

Baba Gagangiri for bringing to my awareness the knowledge that it was a work of lifetimes of rigorous *sadhana* that is culminating in a book in this lifetime.

Master Charles for lending clarity about bringing the experience into the open.

The *yogis* on our plane and those from other realms, for their ongoing help and guidance in my spiritual quest.

My friend Usha Banerji, for being my sounding board on our morning walks.

Dr. Amodini Bagwe for her unstinted guidance, support and constant gentle pushing to see that I put in my best.

Neela Bahl for patiently going through the essays and helping me convey the message in clear and concise manner.

My children Shibani, Nikki, and Gautam for their gentleness and patience in bearing up with my absorption and obsession for things 'mystical'.

Rohit Arya for listening to me with understanding and giving the whole experience a wider perspective.

Gautam, without whose patience and intervention the book would not have become a reality.

Girish Jathar and Sanjay Malandkar for their efforts to bring the book to completion.

PREFACE

The experiences recounted in this book bring to a peak the mystical events associated with the awakening of the *Kundalini* energy as encountered by Santosh in Volumes I and II. Such experiences never 'conclude' as such; they appear spontaneously many times in life after their initial advent. However, this book may represent the culmination of one phase of mystical experience, after which the flow of insight did not take on a predominantly visual form. The forms and scenes encountered by the inner eye become full of clarity and simplicity as well as resonant with spiritual energy. This is as it should be – the later stages of mystical experience are deeper and richer precisely because it comes from a consciousness that is mature and also, to some extent, habituated to the extraordinary. There is more time – and inclination – to ponder instead of to wonder. The illustrations of the workings of the ascending *Kundalini* energy are, as they were in Volume II, unique and unprecedented. The point is worth reiterating. In all the history and all the literature about the *Kundalini,* there has never been anything like this in detail and delineation of the actual processes. This is a large claim, but a valid one.

It is best that you realise this from perusing the book itself but I cannot desist from pointing out something of special interest. From a layperson's point of view, and from the hitherto available literature on the subject, it would seem a reasonable assumption that the awakened *Kundalini* energy ascends from the lower *chakras* to the topmost in linear sequence. One of the great merits of Santosh's book lies in its pointing out that the *chakra* or *chakras* which need activation will be energised first even if it is apparently out of linear sequence. This is of immense significance, as many people spend inordinate amounts of time worrying that the process has gone awry because the 'wrong' *chakra* becomes active. The book is full of such practical experiential wisdom for all those who are on the path of meditation and *Kundalini*. It is also worth emphasising again that another person's experience will never be precisely duplicated in your own meditations, but the book outlines the broad general principles within which you can easily find your specific individual context.

Nowhere is this more clear than in the reaction to the manuscript that came from a practitioner of Peruvian shamanism. It just emphasised the point made in Volume II that these experiences are not Hindu or *yogic* but universal. Indeed, such experiences are almost generic to the mystical tradition, the differences being not in the actual experiences but in interpretations thereof. This is understandable. Humans are inherently complex pattern makers; witness the thousands of languages that evolved over time to serve the common function of speech. *The mystical experience too is a universal inherent human ability of transcendence, but we view it through our filters of culture, language, experience, environment, age and so on ad infinitum.* Peruvian culture and religious beliefs are as far away from India and yoga as can possibly be, but Meera, the Shaman, found so many points of correspondence between the mystical experiences as to confirm the point about universality that I was making above. Her insights and correlations have been presented here as the Afterword and they add an invaluable dimension to this book. As it was, the third volume was full of experiences underwritten by a Universal context; this input by Meera became one of those fortuitous 'coincidences' that always occur in such cases.

On a personal note, I wish to conclude with my own testimony as to the worth of this book. Between Volumes II and III something astonishing happened. My spiritual practices, spotty and sporadic then, caused my own *Kundalini* to awaken and begin its processes. I might add, I was apparently the least likely person this could happen to. Santosh's book was of incalculable value to me in that it clarified many experiences before they could even begin to darken into doubts and fears. The loneliness of the person who has an active *Kundalini* cannot be grasped, for normal people either do not understand or are dismissive. The experiences of Santosh however, were a great map to navigate by. I think I was spared all the natural worry that the sheer enormity of the event engenders, and could just relax and enjoy what was unfolding. There is simply no doubt that Santosh's pioneering work made the path easy for me. My comments on Santosh's illustrations and diary entries are marked with R.A. before the same.

Welcome to the path of transcendence that is the Universal *Kundalini*.

– Rohit Arya

Transitions (From Volume-II)

These pictures recapitulate the classic stages of the spiritual journey. At first, it is a social endeavour with fellow seekers all aiding one another. Then, there is an experience of the personal god, and finally, there is Pure Consciousness albeit not yet the Supreme form of it. This also reiterates the themes running through these books of moving from the purely individual to Universal experiences of the spiritual.

18 September 1996

Evening: I am using my left eye. There is a long procession of people wearing turbans. Some are walking, while others are travelling in bullock carts, atop horses or donkeys, and in all sundry forms of transport. Part of the group on foot is carrying a small, golden palanquin. They climb up a steep, winding path till they come to a golden mountain with a round, open mouth. There is constant movement inside it. The procession of people also disappears inside.

19 September 1996

While meditating in the evening, I see a gigantic, rocky mountain. Through this, a huge lion bursts out with force, along with water, and is charging towards me in slow motion. As he reaches me, I pick up a jug of water and start to pour it into his mouth. I look at the lion as a symbol of *Goddess Durga.*

23 September 1996

I'm on another planet. It is an arid place, devoid of foliage. Then, I step onto a platform of sorts along with a companion. It takes off and we land on a smooth, green expanse. We step down and start walking – where to I don't know. At one stage, there is a concentrated flow of Consciousness, part of which thins out and separates. The concentrated Consciousness gets under the lighter one, divides at the centre, and then both merge into each other. This happens in between the states of stillness.

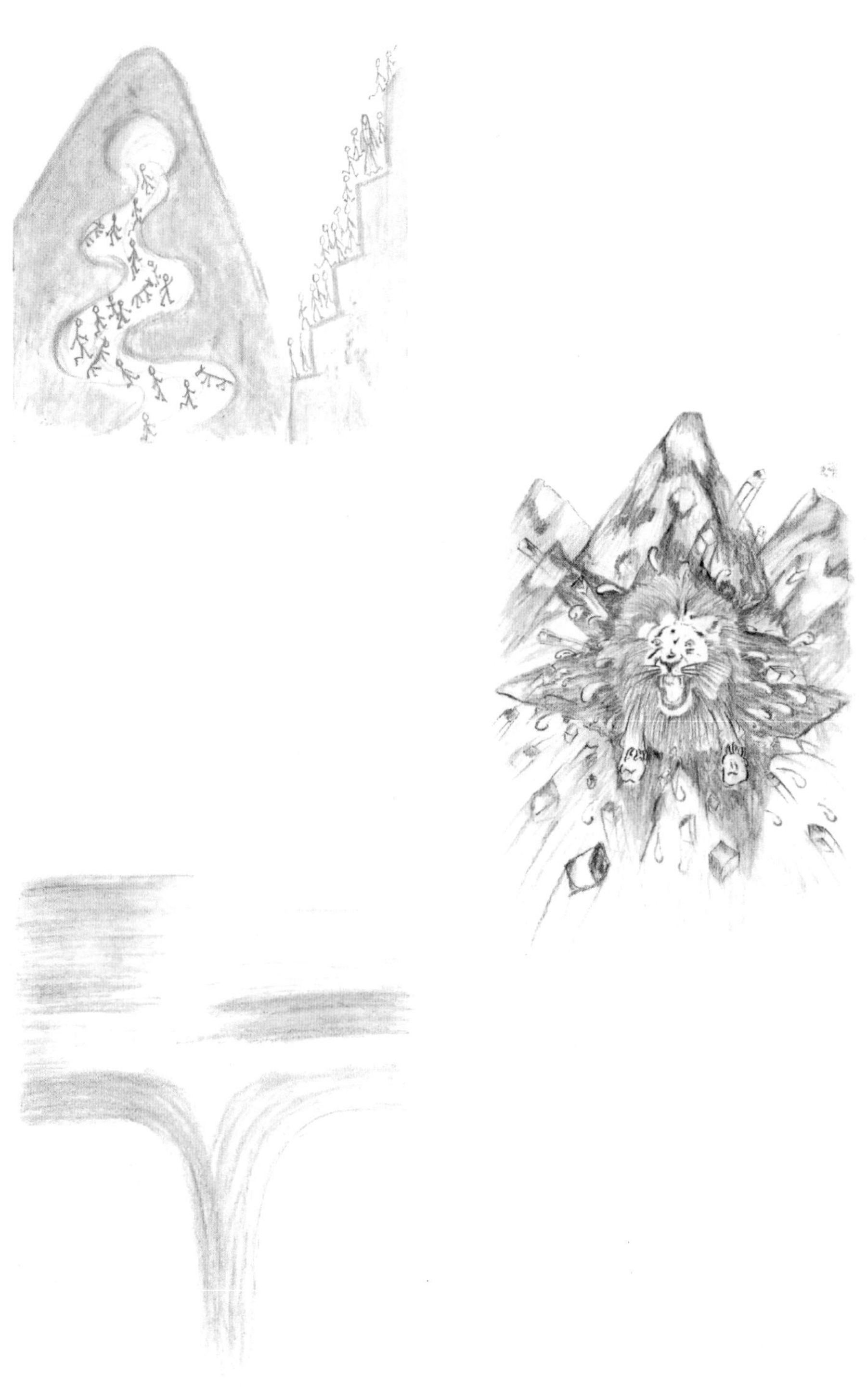

AFFIRMATION

I am now entering upon the greatest teaching accessible to man, for I am learning the secret of existence.

The riddle of the universe is about me; I am now solving it.

I learn why men die, why they are born, and why they live.

I learn why men succeed and why they fail, why they are happy and why they are discontent. I have the power and the ability to live as long as I desire, to achieve whatever I wish, and the doors of my mind are now open that I may learn how this is done.

I now learn that man is the master of his destiny, that man is the author of his death. I realise that death is a mental concept and not a law of life.

I now realise that all negation is a mental concept and not a law of life.

I learn that there is only one law of creation – the law of life.

I am now developing the power and the ability to realise in my own life the one divine principle in which all success, happiness, and peace reside.

And I thank the Infinite Spirit within me
For the knowledge of this wondrous truth
Now revealed to my consciousness.

– Ramanathan, Swami K. S. – 'Mental Physics: Lectures and Lessons'. (Private circulation), Bombay, India, 1980, p. 142.

"A snake came to my water-trough...
Being earth-brown, earth-golden from the burning
bowels of the earth...
But must I confess how I liked him,
How glad I was he had come like a guest in quiet,
to drink at my water-trough
And depart peaceful, pacified and thankless,
Into the burning bowels of this earth?
Was it cowardice, that I dared not kill him?
Was it perversity that I longed to talk to him?
Was it humility, to feel so honoured?
I felt so honoured...
For he seemed to me again like a king,
Like a king in exile, uncrowned in the underworld,
Now due to be crowned again."

Snake
– D. H. Lawrence

INTRODUCTION

This is the third book in the series pertaining to the awakening of *Kundalini* and subsequent insights gained.

This is a new way of understanding how the body-mind intellect moves/works towards actualising its thought, wish, or desire; the process of actualising and manifesting is set in motion as soon as the conscious thought occurs. Just as when the food reaches the stomach the process of digestion starts, in the same way, actualisation of the wish is also programmed into the system. And, just as when we put different foods into the stomach at one given time we are heading towards indigestion and discomfort, in the same manner, if we pile up too many requests at one time it is going to lead to a haphazard fructification of the results and probably when not required.

The visual experience that these books illustrate serves a dual purpose.

1. It leads me through the step by step purification and changes that had to be brought forth in the body-mind intellect in order to actualise the knowledge I had asked for. This makes me very conscious of the fact that 'I am the master of my destiny and the author of my death'. It literally means that I can have my life and death designed the way I want. The catch lies in the level of my 'awareness' at all times.

2. For the aspirants on the road to self-discovery, this visual journey serves as a point of reference and helps them move along at a faster pace without getting into uncertainties and fears of a different nature.

As the human consciousness expands, the Masters have thought it fit, and the time appropriate, for the experience to come out as a visual journey in order to serve as a guide.

It was only at a late stage that realisation dawned as to what was transpiring. I had expressed a desire to know the origin of my Source. This desire was expressed most casually, not realising that as soon as I made the wish the machinery of my body and mind would be set in motion to give me exactly what I had asked for. Not only that, I was given visual knowledge of the intricacy involved in creating a balance between the emotional, physical, and mental bodies. To ensure that nothing was missed, my awareness remained at an optimum level. This made me very conscious of the fact that I was not just a random speck of creation floating around in the universe, but a focus point of the Source Consciousness, ever alert to my each thought, word, and deed. How could it be possible to give 100% of Itself to every particle of its creation? I came to the realisation that it is possible only if the Source is residing within me. As balance was brought about in the negative and positive polarities, the subtle dimension of Witness Consciousness opened up.

In order to manifest the experience, the three books contain all the visuals related to the changes, with corresponding knowledge that the mental, physical, and emotional bodies had to go through. I list a few of the main ones:

Volume I: P. 44, 45, 63 – activation of the *Ajna chakra;* purification of *Prana.* P. 48, 56, 60 – balancing left and right cortical regions or the negative and positive polarities. P. 53, 75 – cleansing of the subtle bodies. P. 80, 102, 132, 179 – activating and synchronising the *chakras.* P. 104 – awakening of *Kundalini.*

Volume II: P. 43 – third eye given the ability to survey the inner as well as the outer subtle dimensions. P. 51, 65 – moving through regions of memory and outer dimensions. P. 57 – expansion of consciousness. P. 89 – destruction of the old psyche. P. 131 – consciousness in recognition of itself. P. 151, 157 – erasing and inscribing – creating new grooves in the brain. P. 185 – Source Consciousness fragments itself in multi-dimensional experience, thus forfeiting holistic awareness.

Such a complex wish took only five years for manifestation and integration; I realise that if we are focused in our day to day living, we would be creating miracles for ourselves all the time.

Chapter One

I AM – I AM NOT

I have this inherent quality of accepting and believing what is said, with the result that I experienced great excitement and inner joy on reading the lines, *"I am now entering upon the greatest teaching accessible to man, for I am learning the secret of existence...."* It was a very pleasant feeling to have, and to know, that in order to access the 'secret of existence', what I was required to do was to be regular in my practice of the breathing exercises and affirmations and the rest would unfold for me through my meditations. I took this for granted.

I soon realised that it was not as simple as I believed, but that a process had to be set in operation, which would get my body-mind intellect functioning to the required vibratory level or frequency in order to solve 'the riddle of the universe'. The first book visualises mainly the cleansing of the etheric body with the gentle movement of *Kundalini*. The second book shows the result of the cleansing and restructuring of the grooves in the brain, along with shattering the old and creating the new psyche. I do some astral travel and visit different planes, encountering along the way the adventures related to that vibratory level. I move back in my memory and visualise scenes from different lives that help me understand my hopes and fears and know myself better. I get to know and absorb the meaning of the *Guru* principle, and finally acknowledge my experience as an experience in Consciousness. When I say 'I', it is not the 'I' as in body consciousness, but the 'I' as formless Consciousness.

9 October 1996

The time had now come when the physical body had to be taken care of before I could move ahead in an endeavour to know my Source. This care was going to be taken up by the Masters who were supervising my unfoldment from another realm. I am eternally grateful to them for their sensitivity, love, and care. I am also required to put my attention to some serious study of the solar system. We are pouring over some maps, but I prove to be an inattentive student, testing the patience of the Masters. However, with their constant guidance and help, in due course, I learnt to move and experiment on my own.

With the enthusiasm to transcend different vibratory levels at a fast pace, I encounter a barrier which, in spite of putting in all my effort, I am unable to surmount; it is as though I am trying to push against an attic door. With persistent trying, I manage to create a slit, through which I get a glimpse of blinding, white light. Was I trying to get past the Crown *chakra*?

> *"The Divine Light comes not through open doors but only through narrow slits. The aspirant sees the ray as a sunbeam passing through a chink into a dark room. It is like a 'flash of lightning'."*
>
> *– Sivananda, Swami – 'Concentration and Meditation'. The Divine Life Society, U.P., India. Eighth Edition, 1990, p. 323.*

However, after this futile attempt, it seemed necessary that my gross body goes through some sort of surgery by the Masters in the astral realm. This is one area where outside help is required, and the *Kundalini* energy needed this passage to be cleared for her, for whatever the blockage here, it had probably become too gross. The blockages that the energy has to clear in its path before it can move smoothly, are related to the emotional and mental blocks pertaining to love, hate, jealousy, resentment, fear, pride, mistrust, and guilt, which get solidified over a period of time and settle as deposits in different parts of the body, if not resolved and dissolved.

It is likely that my brain and my heart are not synchronising; there is an in-built clash between emotions and rigid attitudes or value systems; some fixed ideas of right and wrong. These became solidified and settled in the physical heart region. *Kundalini* could clear the *chakras* and the meridians in the etheric body but the gross body needed to be taken care of and the blocks removed in order to render the process effective. This could also happen through meditation, but the process would be slow and time consuming. Care is also taken to see that there is no wear or tear in the *aura* in order to render me absolutely safe from outside influences as and when consciousness moves out of the physical body, thus leaving it unattended.

10 October 1996

4:30 am: The energy starts to rise from the base of the spine and travels up on the right side of the body, fully energising it, giving a certain tingling sensation. It then starts to spread to the left side of the body, till the whole body is fully charged with energy. A tube inside the upper part of the body begins to extend, and another one approaches it from the outer space. Both clamp together at the navel, to be gradually drawn out and away. This is perhaps the Guide Consciousness leading the Individual Consciousness to explore the astral dimensions.

I am surrendered to the forces of transformation in the course of the meditation, and willingly submit to the seemingly tortuous process even though I don't understand it at all. I am simply a detached observer. A long, wooden pole is thrust into my chest with a thud, which gives me a jerk like a massive jolt of electric shock. The energy starts flowing around the pole and, in quick succession, I cross two vibratory levels.

12 October 1996
(Nadi Replacement Surgery)

There is a great pressure on my feet, more on the left foot. Then, a tube with a magnet at its end is lowered into my chest with keen concentration and precision (Fig. 1). Another instrument follows it, and it does its job of scraping and cleaning an artery.

A small, round-toothed disc is released, which travels up the chest towards the throat (Fig. 2 & 3). The lever pulls up the instrument inserted earlier into the chest. Attached to it is another length of tube. As it is completely extracted from the chest, the nut and bolt, or the magnet, are discarded (Fig. 4). I notice that light is being thrown from behind the head across the full length of the body, like in an operation theatre.

Evening meditation: A gadget is heated and lowered into the chest to seal the wound. For this purpose heat and light is used instead of sutures.

10:30 pm: On putting my head to the pillow, I immediately see dark red (almost black) blood starting to drip from the chest on to the floor. I see small black insects crawling in it. When the phenomenon does not stop on its own, I ask it to stop. It stops dripping, and the vision comes to an end.

Fig. 1

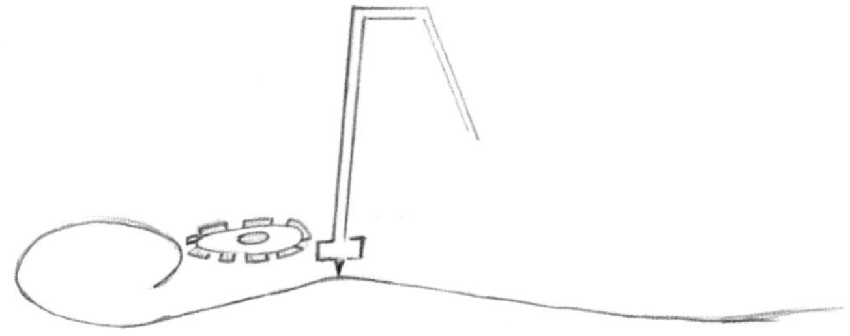

Fig. 2

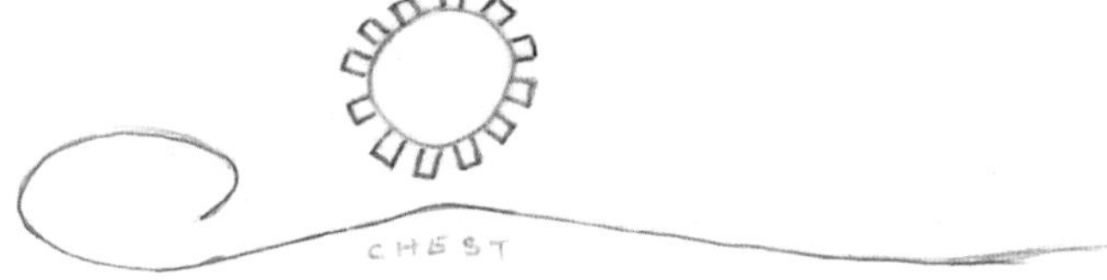

Fig. 3

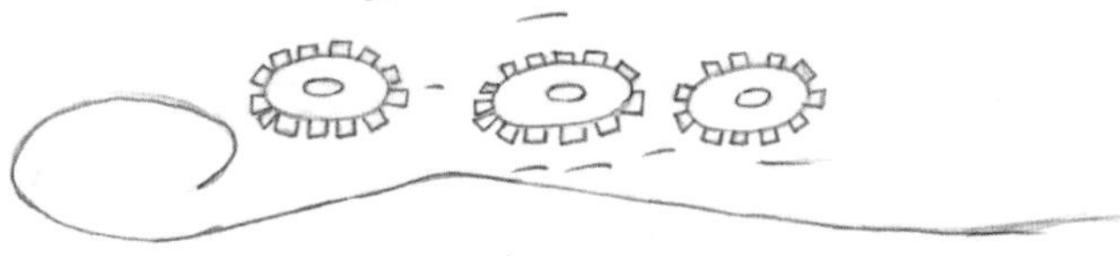

Fig. 4

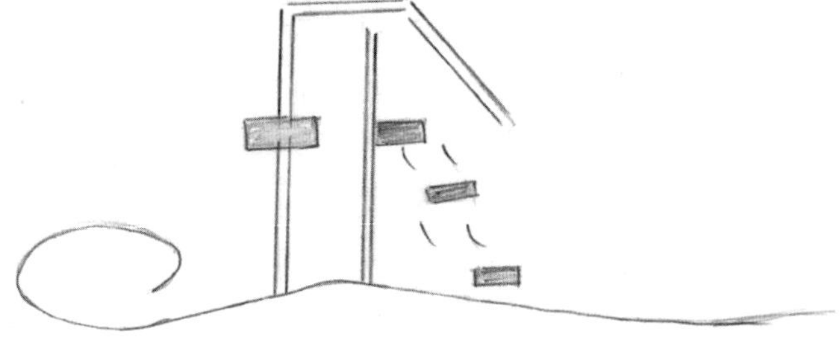

14 October 1996

Evening: Good after-care is rendered during meditation or while sleeping. I am given some dark liquid to drink from a decorative spoon.

15 October 1996

4:30 am: People from all walks of life are going around me doing *pradakshina* or circumambulation (going around me in circles), and then are backing away from me with a look of veneration, as though I am an idol in a temple. I realise that this is yet another instance of identification with the Cosmic Consciousness.

16 October 1996

I'm in the realm of flowers. There are beautiful flowers of different colours, varieties, and fragrances. Then I see what appears like a *Shivalinga,* encircled by a dull yellow snake. Slowly, the *Shivalinga* starts rotating along with the golden snake encircling it. Both become one colour, radiating golden light. The *Shivalinga* catches speed and starts submerging in a whirlpool, until it disappears. What remains is the rippling surface of water.

> R. A.: The golden *linga* seems to be a *Jyotirlinga,* the famed *linga* of light. That it disappears into water is not surprising. *Jyotirlingas* tend to do that once the purpose for which they have manifested is over.

"According to the science of tantra, kundalini and yoga, there are twelve places in the physical body where shivalingam is located in the same shape. Out of those twelve, three are considered very important. One is in mooladhara chakra (swayambhulingam), the second in ajna chakra (itaralingam) and the third in sahasrara chakra (paralingam). It is said that in sahasrara chakra the finest consciousness resides in the shape of an illuminated shivalingam."

– Muktibodhananda, Swami – 'Hatha Yoga Pradipika'. Yoga Publication Trust, Munger, Bihar, India, 1985. Reprinted, 2000, p. 533.

"As in the supreme state She lay coiled as the Mahakundali round the Supreme Siva..."

– Woodroffe, Sir John – 'The Serpent Power'. Ganesh & Company, Madras, India. First Paperback Edition, 1995, p. 41.

In the evening meditation, a finger makes three crosses (x x x) across my right thigh. The action is repeated as if to make sure that I register it. The focus on it made me very apprehensive, and I seemed to conclude that it was some sort of warning of an accident related to my leg. This same leg has been through accidents in other lifetimes.

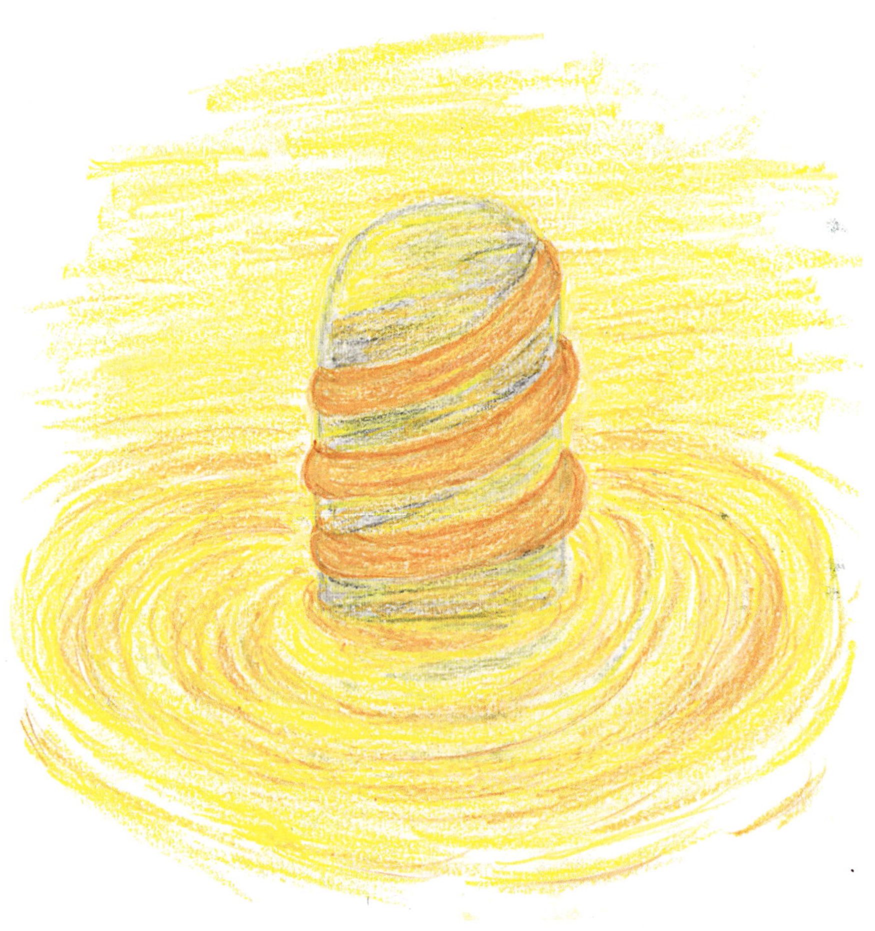

17 October 1996

During meditation, I am being shown a chart containing certain symbols and constellations. There is a finger pointing here and there. My attention is not focused, and I don't comprehend. The Masters lose patience and, in annoyance, the chart is taken away. Then, a youthful figure with a big head of curly hair catches hold of my hand and makes me sit close to him. He starts to talk to me intensely, but I still don't comprehend a thing. Then suddenly, doors open and I realise that I must enter. I go as consciousness, but I am a transparent body. I become the void with its continuous resonating *nada* (sound of the unbeaten drum). Off and on, I see with me the curly head floating around, also transparent. I realise that it is Sathya Sai Baba. Then I start coming together and form a transparent hollow globe in the void. The whole process has been initiated with the activation of the Heart *chakra,* with a shift to the Navel *chakra,* and then to the ears.

Afternoon: After-care to the surgery still continues from the astral realm. While resting after lunch, one half of a small tablet is pressed on my tongue.

17 October 1996

Evening: I meditate to a devotional music cassette. I see a whole lot of people clapping and swaying to the music. As the music ends, a stray, unclean looking dog comes and lies down at a little distance from me. I go to see if it is hurt. Instead, there is a *rishi* who is quite robust. In front of my eyes he is transformed into a starved looking, bent, bearded old *Sadhu*. I kneel down and prostrate myself at his feet, begging forgiveness for being inattentive earlier. I attribute the bedraggled state of the sage to the disrespect I have shown him earlier by not making the effort to learn what I am being taught. I then find myself in a cave with the sages sitting around. I am dancing the *tandav* as a woman. There is a dark oval shape over my head. I can't tell whether it is my hair flying up as I dance, or snakes, or what. I see vibrations as tiny red flames fluttering on my chest.

18 October 1996

A *chakra* is coming at great speed from the outer space. It stops over my chest, to the right. It keeps rotating and gently descending till it moves into the chest. It acts on a *nadi* (artery) with a blockage. The blockage is blown off with the force of the energy. It is quite fascinating to watch how different methods are being adopted to clear my blocked *nadis* in the physical body, so that the energy can move more freely and I can fulfil the purpose of my being. It brings to my mind the words from the Bible, "Ask and you shall receive, knock and it shall be opened unto you." I have been asking the Source to reveal the purpose of my being, and it seems I am getting the answer now, even though the Almighty has to put me on to the operating table to hasten the process in order to realise my purpose in this life itself.

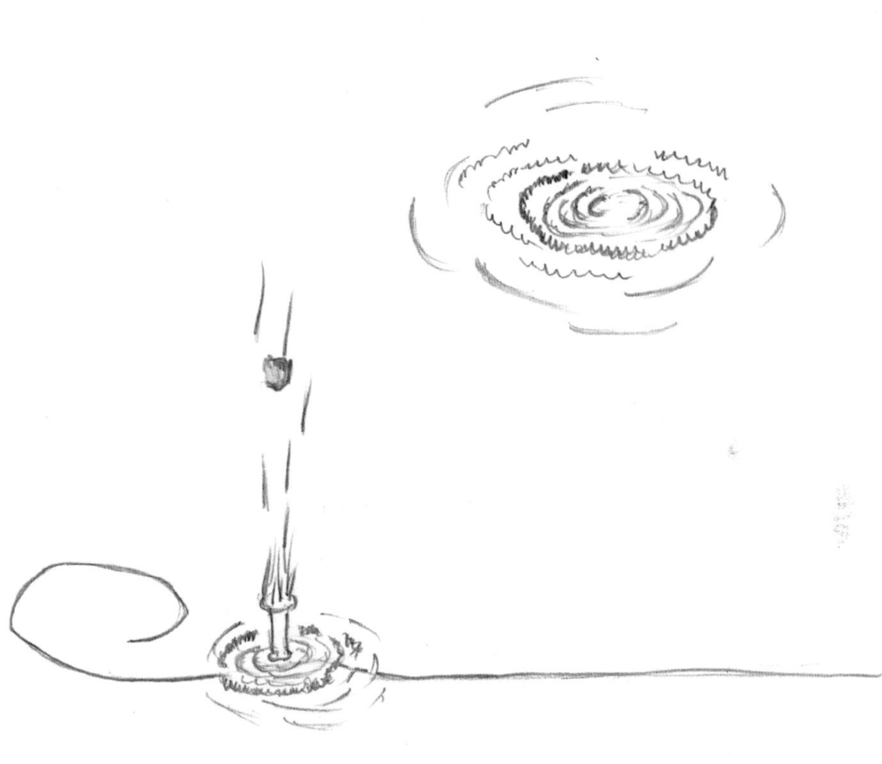

20 October 1996

A door opens on the right side of my body and I enter as consciousness. Only part of the consciousness is allowed in, and the door closes.

22 October 1996

The sensation in the feet continues, more so in the left foot. At one point, I see a big wheel rotating over my feet. The left foot and the *chakra* in the right temple seem to be connected. There is adjustment in the right temple *chakra*. It is set in motion and then stopped at a certain angle. Vibrations are set off in the left temple and, in order to synchronise or control the vibration, a transparent white band, almost like a band aid, is put to balance the *chakra* in the left temple (as if repairing a damaged *chakra*) or to hold it together at a certain angle.

I'm focused in the heart and it seems I'm in a field of golden corn.

A globe is rotating in the air, and there is a big hole in it. Every time the hole passes my vision, I get a blinding glimpse of white light.

Moving in the clouds, I find myself in a white palace that has no walls. I am sitting at a white, ornate dining table laid with white, ornate cutlery and crockery. I sense another presence; I am served breakfast.

23 October 1996

4:30 am: I am standing in a temple. The bells are moving of their own accord. I see myself in saffron robes at the rear end of the temple. Who is the watcher, then? Do I see myself or is it my consciousness, slowly moving backwards until the door closes?

7:30 am: Today, during meditation, the mind stopped. I experienced total non-functioning of the mind and lack of awareness. Consciousness is focused in the heart region. Then, flashes of fire start going out of the head. The head suddenly jerks when consciousness or awareness returns. There is a feeling of water dripping from the tips of the fingers; it is so real that I open my eyes to look.

24 October 1996

I cannot go through the affirmations. The mind is not functioning. At one stage, a glow is radiating from the abdomen in an upward direction towards the chest, and there is a sensation of warmth, indicating that the energy has moved up to the level of the *Manipur chakra,* and is spreading its shining *aura* above and beyond the body.

25 October 1996

Awareness lapsed off and on, indicating that I was floating between, and moving in and out of a very deep level in the course of the meditation.

26 October 1996

I realise how hard it is to subdue the mind. No matter how alert I try to stay, it stealthily tries to get back in control. I now seem to know its nature. I have learnt not to fight the mind; I've learnt to let it be alone and not to interfere with whatever it brings up. If it still distracts me, then it is fine, and I realise that I can do both things simultaneously, i.e. meditate as well as watch the thoughts. It is very interesting.

27 October 1996

The energy first moved through the left side of the body and made it complete. It made me feel that my left side was whole. Then it went through the right side of the body, giving me the same feeling. They are, in fact, two complete bodies. The consciousness gathers together and starts moving out of the right temple, and into a tunnel. It goes on and on until it gets completely sucked out, and what remains is a body of light. What went out? What remained? What came back? The head jerks as consciousness returns.

Energy moved from the heart to the head, and then out. I am just a void in motion... I am such a vast void in a peaceful, slow, rhythmic, spiral motion, winding and unwinding.

> R. A.: To feel herself as a spiral motion in the void is somewhat more remarkable than it seems, for the spiral is Nature's perfect shape. Even galaxies instinctively align themselves so as to avoid the burnout that would come many millennia earlier, were they not configured so. The spiral is about the only natural form that is in a dynamic state of unstable equilibrium. Spirals are the natural curve of life and uniform growth; yet they never go over the same ground. Also, a spiral is the only type of curve where different parts differ in size, not shape. Spirals alone, amongst curved lines, can be extended infinitely. They are *yin yang*, order in chaos, opposites that are not so; they are magic. Even Aikido, the most philosophical and profound of all the martial arts, used the spiral as the basis of all breath and creativity. The founder of the system, Morehei Uyeshiba, was somewhat of a monomaniac about the body-psyche-spiral connection. Santosh's realisation is part of that universal understanding.

In the evening, I find that the *Ajna chakra* is straining to meet the *Anahat chakra.*

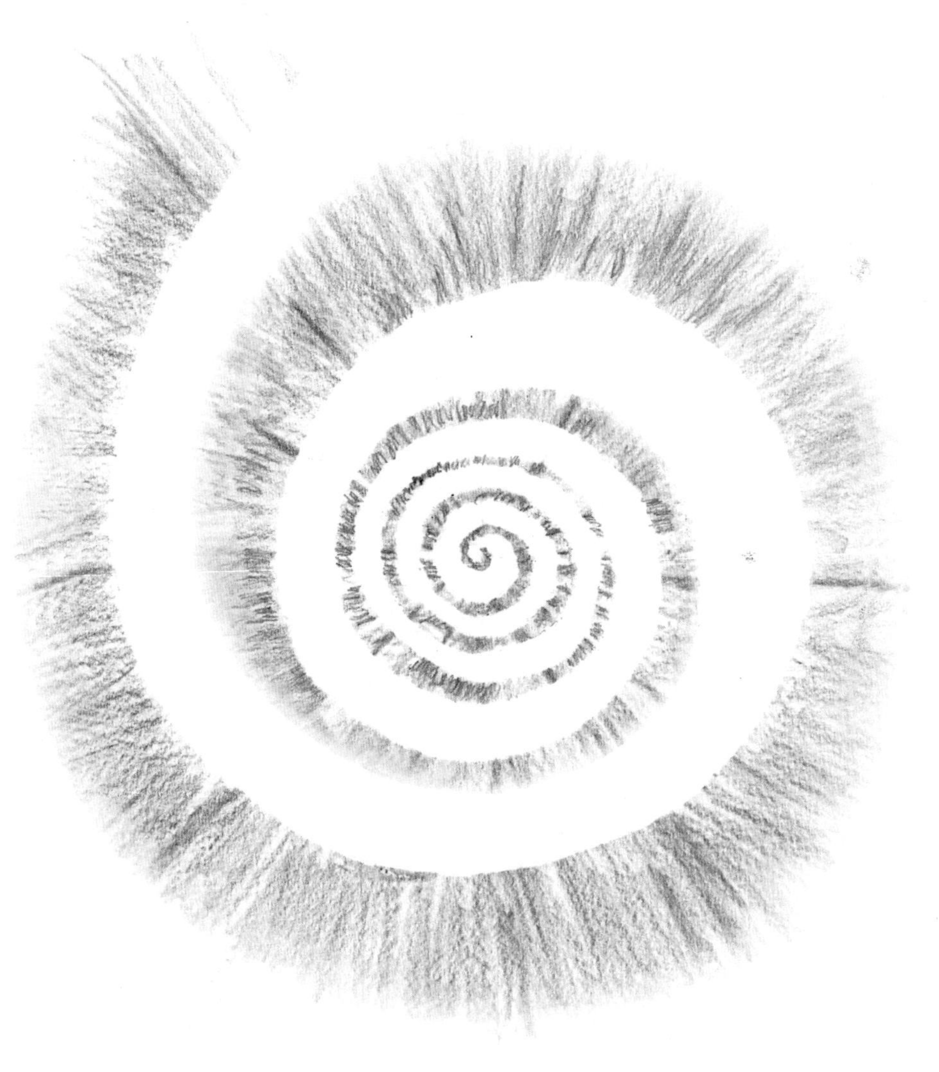

1 November 1996

4:30 am: I see *devas* in shining attire with gold embroidered cloth belts around their tunics and wearing close fitting crowns, marching into my chest.

2 November 1996

4:30 am: The whole body is in a flux. I wonder if I will ever be able to move as a whole organism again. Later, there is a jerk at the base of the spine as consciousness returns to the body.

7:30 am: Soft, misty-coloured energy is focused at the eye level. It begins entering through the eyes, and then moves out of the eyes. There is the sensation of the eyes moving with the *Prana.*

13 November 1996

I see different instruments being used to repair my *aura*. An etching needle is tracing smooth curves and loops upon it (Fig. 1). A tiny, round ball with a rod for a handle is used to smoothen the creases in the *aura;* and the etching needle moves efficiently. I am aware that my *aura* is being repaired in a required manner (Fig. 2). Also, a gadget like an X-ray machine is scanning the body by throwing light and moving over the body, almost like a scanner (Fig. 3).

"When an unreconstructed personality tries to resist Kundalini, consciously or unconsciously, She may fry nerves and blow out endocrine fuses, shorting out the nervous system at its weakest point and blowing a hole in the victim's aura. Since the aura's job is to insulate us psychically from one another and from disembodied influences, holes in the aura permit all sorts of chaotic, negative mental vibrations, including even ethereal parasites, to enter the individual's field as they like and spread ruin."

– Svoboda, Robert E. – 'Kundalini Aghora II'. Rupa & Co., Calcutta, India, 1993. Third Impression, 1996, p. 58.

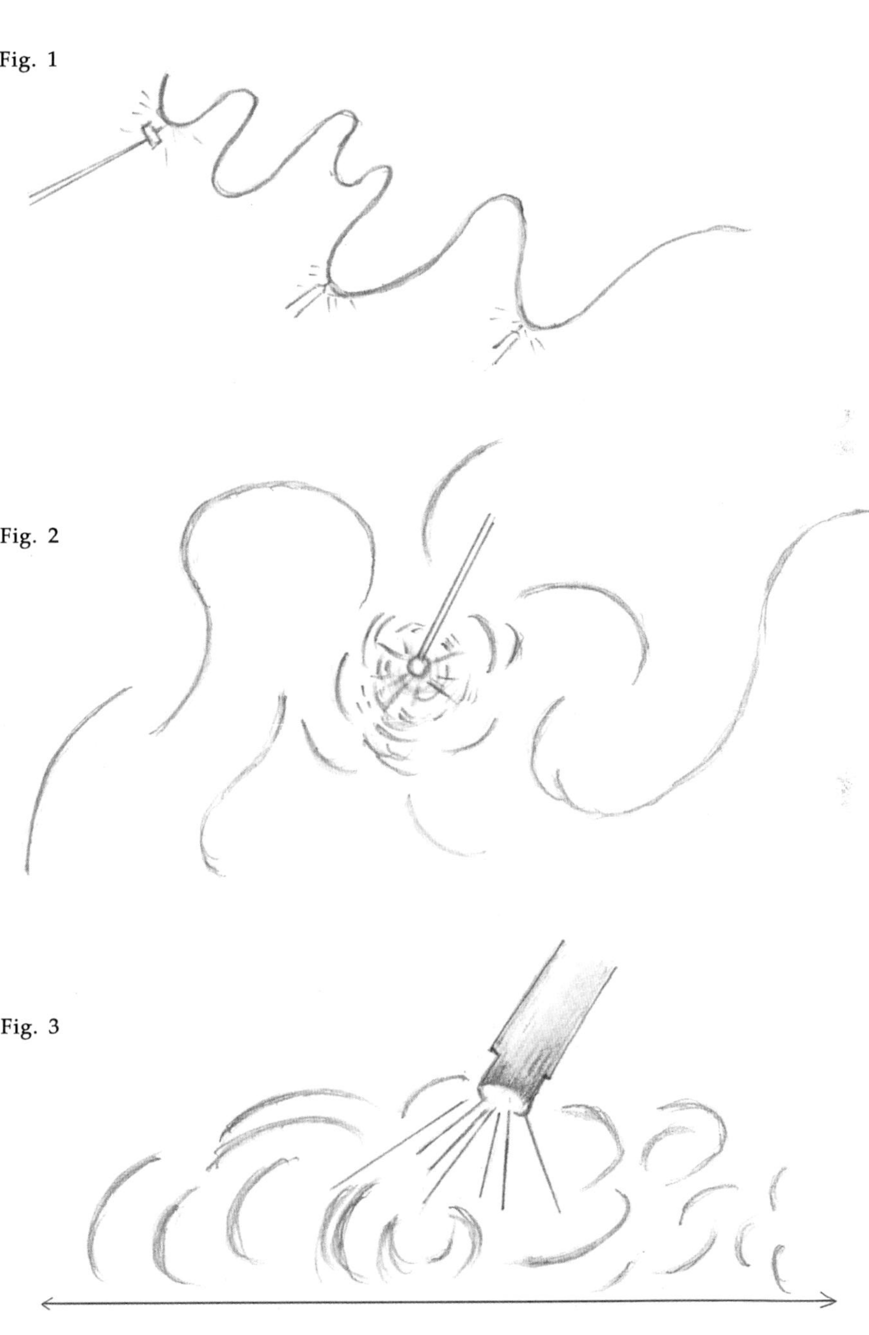
Fig. 1
Fig. 2
Fig. 3

14 November 1996

Evening meditation: The etheric body seems to be making preparations for another phase. There is pressure of energy in the left jaw, pushing it further to the left. Then, the same is repeated in the right jaw. The area where the neck joins the jaw also experiences a constriction. The breathing is strained. I then feel a plug-like object being pushed up my palate, with the result that the area above is lighted up, and it throws up sparks of light which trigger a *chakra* in the right temple.

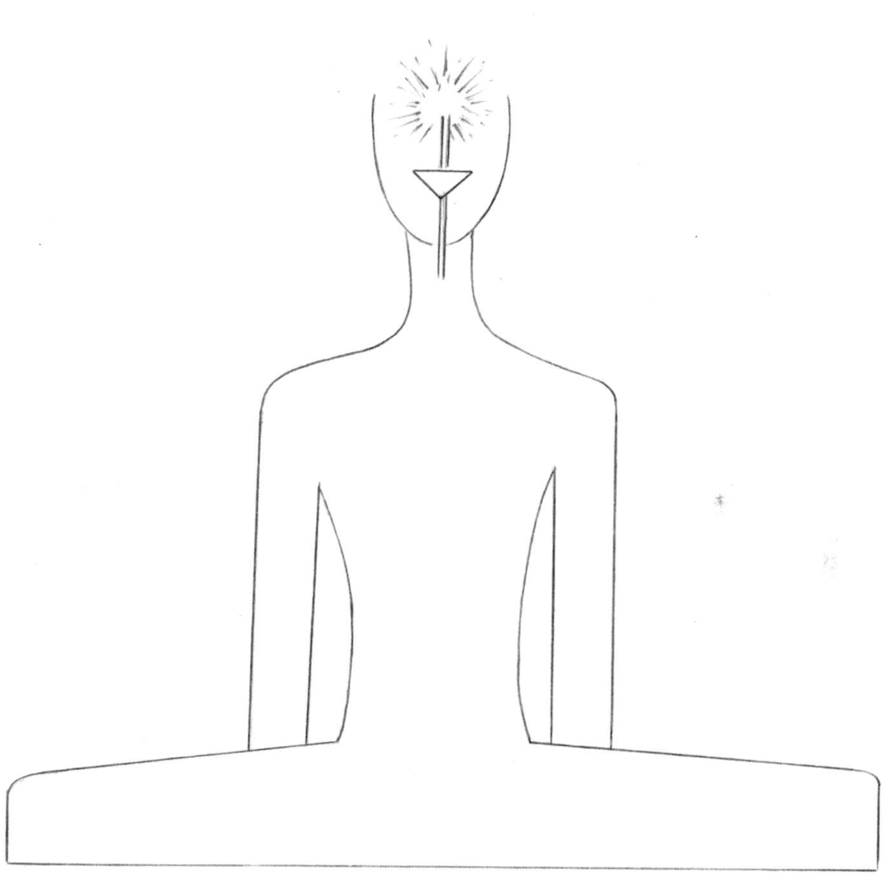

20 November 1996

We went to Khopoli (outside Mumbai) to visit Baba Gagangiri at his ashram. The trip proved essential for my spiritual growth.

21 November 1996

A white glow rises from the chest towards the face. During meditation, from the chest upwards, there is the feeling of a forceful *Prana* pushing and propelling me at considerable speed in a straight course, seemingly for eons and eons. There is no more meandering, and I shoot out like a rocket. I don't reach anywhere in particular. Somehow, I feel like *Hanuman.*

"The element of wind, which flows upto the navel of physical body, has a curved way of flowing. The wind is circulating within the body in 49 various ways, and these cause the waves in mind or disturbances in mind... Shri Guru straightens the crooked flow of these Vayus, and one by one, virtues begin to develop."

– Ashish – 'The Eternal Culture of the Masters'. Shree Gagangiri Prakashan, Khopoli, India, July 1995, p. 151.

22 November 1996

Thanks to Baba Gagangiri, speed seems to be the essence at this stage in my meditation. I continue moving through different tunnels at terrific speed. This must be the *Kundalini* working in the intricate passages in the brain cortex.

Evening: Another door closed today. This is the third such door closing in the last fortnight.

"When you arouse Kundalini before your mind is firmly under control, She will very likely self-identify even more strongly with your limitations, which can wreak havoc with your evolutionary progress. A good Guru will close the doors to the lowest three chakras so that the Kundalini can never fall back into them. Then there is very little danger; otherwise the disciple will be most likely overwhelmed with the desire for food, sleep, or sex."

– Svoboda, op. cit., p. 67.

26 November 1996

From an inch above the navel, a knot, the size of a pea, gets pushed up with each breath till it arrives just below the ribs. At some stage, I see the energy as a shining, small, dark ball, the size of a pea, bouncing around at random, between the heart and the navel.

27 November 1996

An explosion goes off in the head, shaking my whole body.

2 December 1996

Extending from the temples is a straight and long tunnel.

The *Ajna chakra* gets active. The vibrations of the *chakra* create wings in front of the forehead, and then at the sides of the temples. It seems I am preparing for a big flight to another dimension.

There is expansion from the *Spleen chakra.* I experience discomfort and distension in the abdomen; the body starts expanding.

Every day, off and on during the meditations, there are flashes of people talking to me. I understand what they are saying. Mainly, I am listening and nodding my head. Even though I don't speak, they seem to comprehend my answers. *Guruji* tells me that here the communication is at a different level. It is done through 'thought'.

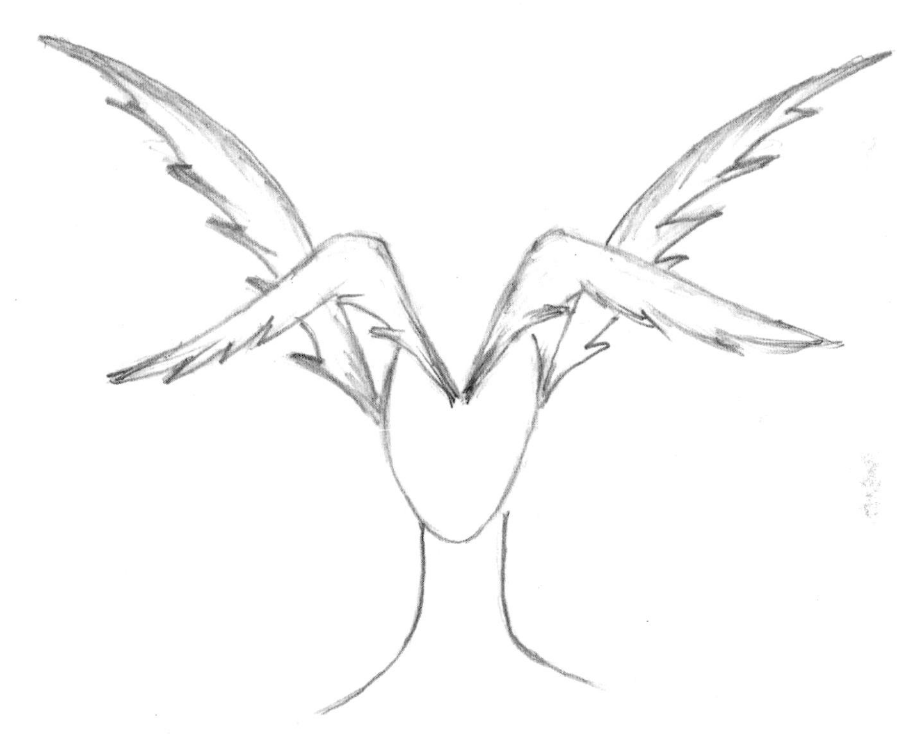

4 December 1996

Just as the body is gross, there is density in consciousness also. At different levels of density, it experiences the phenomena at that level.

When I am helped out of the body, my own consciousness is rather dense, while that of the guide is a rarefied consciousness, so that I need support to keep afloat in order to travel to the rarefied astral dimensions. The guide initiates adjustment to facilitate smooth and free movement.

I learn that as consciousness rises to higher planes it tends to become more rarefied, and it becomes denser and turns into matter while descending to the earthly plane. But, in order to move at all, whether to rise higher or to go to the nether dimensions, it has to match the vibratory pattern and level of that dimension.

4 December 1996

Now, with sufficient experience in astral travel in the course of my meditations, my consciousness is so rarefied that I move with freedom without any hindrance or resistance.

Earlier, when I was still a novice and my system was not tuned, while crossing a vibratory level, I knew I was switching dimensions because of a difference in the vibration pattern which would even out when I was fully into the next vibratory plane. This shift, or movement, would remind me of a car going over rumbling speed breakers. Now, with greater mastery over management of the consciousness in flight, there is achieved, somehow, a better attunement between a vibratory motion of each plane/ dimension and the consciousness, so that the transitions are smooth, almost unnoticeable. Only at the highest planes (from my perspective) there may be slight disturbance in the form of a gentle ripple marking such a journey or a shift in consciousness.

4 December 1996

I see a grinder rotating and it emits splinters of light upon catching momentum. This image often accompanies the experience of being stuck between two astral vibratory levels, or if I have reached a point of stagnation in meditation. All I need to do, however, is to invoke the *Guru,* to bring forth a sense of release and smooth passage to the next level of experience.

> R. A.: This recurring image is very significant for it recalls a famous couplet by one of India's greatest mystics, Kabir.
>
> *Chalti chaakki dekh ke, diya Kabira roye*
> *Do paatan ke beech mein, sabith bacha na koye.*
>
> (*Seeing the two grindstones move, Kabir wept –*
> *For nothing survives between the millstones*)
>
> It is an appalling metaphor for the dreary inevitability of the unaware life. Santosh is clear that the vision comes to her only in moments of 'stuckness' and she needs her *Guru's* grace to push past it. Even Kabir, great Master though he was, had quailed before the grimness of the vision.

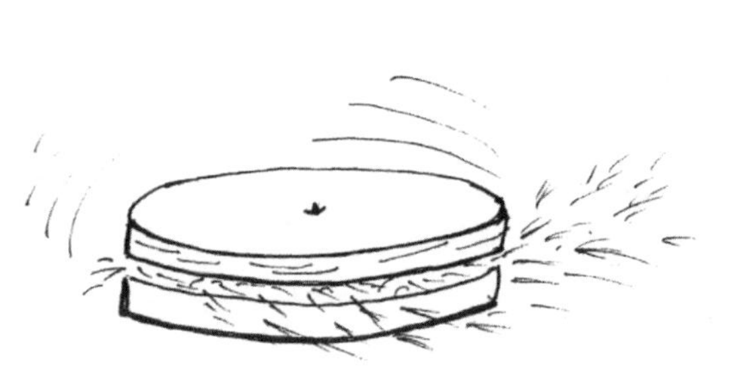

5 December 1996

While travelling in one particular dimension, I see beings of solid, white light, with dark, round eyes. Now and then, one of them comes at a tremendous speed, brushes across my ears with a sharp sound of *whoosh* and disappears. The sensation of energy concentrated in the big toe of the left foot continues.

"These divine bodies of similar type have no Yonis or genetive organs but were illuminated souls. The movements were all based so speedily much more forceful than microwaves. The golden light was so satisfying and blissful that everyone would freely stay there permanently. This is the 'Tattwa Darshan'."

– Patel, Dadubhai N. – 'The Real Essence of Tantra'. Yogi Divine Society, Bombay, India, 1978, p. 195.

"These august Beings have been called the Lords of the Flame and the Children of the Fire-mist, and They have produced a wonderful effect upon our evolution. The intellect of which we are so proud is almost entirely due to Their presence, for in the natural course of events the next round, the fifth, should be that of intellectual advancement... and such advance is entirely due to the assistance given by these great Lords of the Flame. Most of Them stayed with us only through that critical period of our history; a few still remain to hold the highest offices of the Great White Brotherhood..."

– Leadbeater, C. W. – 'A Text Book of Theosophy'. The Theosophical Publishing House, Adyar, India, 1912. Fourteenth Reprint, 1997, pp. 131-132.

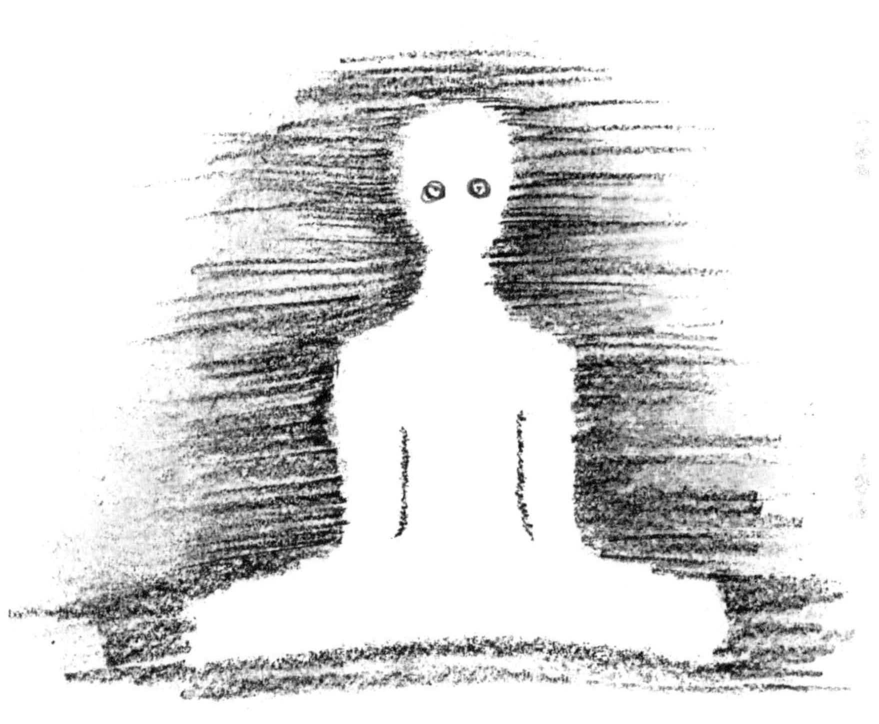

6 December 1996

I see two hazy discs hovering close together over the length of my body like a dead weight. They look like the two parts of the grinder, only now they are parallel to each other, hovering over my body. As they move apart there is a feeling of expansion, and as soon as my awareness wavers they come back together. I make them move as far apart as possible, with a conscious effort, and the sensation of expansion increases. I lose that and then the left temple is a splash of light with a yellow centre (reminding me of a fried egg with sunny side up). It starts moving out and expanding. It comes back in the shape of a boomerang.

There is a big thump on the chest as if someone had hit me with the flat of the palm, perhaps to ease the way out of being stuck or shock me out of a certain vibratory level. The whole body vibrates with the thump.

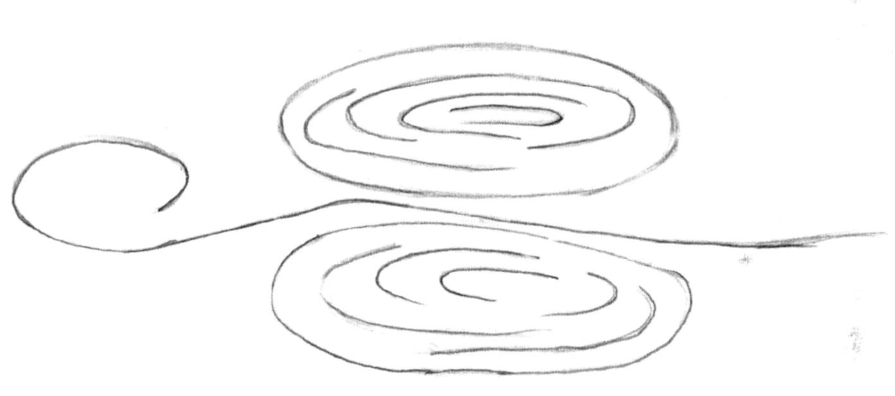

12 December 1996

I feel totally free. Love, life, and joy freely flow to me from all directions. I am left with a sense of buoyancy and euphoria, which I want to share with all.

7:30 am: Though there is a sense of freedom i.e. I no longer feel stuck during meditation, there is heaviness in the left foot, with a corresponding heaviness in the right side of the chest, below the collarbone and towards the shoulders, extending downwards. The energy in the head is being slowly pulled down towards the chest, creating a vacuum in the head. (Is this the death of the mind?) It barely reaches down, when it starts moving outwards and expanding. A bubble of energy starts moving from the base of the spine upwards, in the right side of the body.

14 December 1996

I am This and I am That. I am stillness and I am also movement.

Even as meditation 'just happens', initiation to establish a relationship with the divine is also a very spontaneous event. I now understand why it is said that "the *Guru* will manifest when the student is ready." Usually, the Master-Disciple relationship continues life after life, with the Master picking up the threads of the Individual Consciousness wherever they were left off earlier.

16 December 1996

4:30 am: The *Spleen chakra* is fully active. With the activation of the *Spleen chakra* it seems the expansion of the etheric body has started. Earlier, the consciousness left the body behind and went on astral travels, whereas now it takes off in an expansion of wholeness rather than fragmentation. This lends a great sense of euphoria.

"When the second of the etheric centres, that at the spleen, is awakened, the man is enabled to remember his vague astral journeys, though sometimes only very partially."

– Leadbeater, C. W. – 'The Chakras: A Monograph'. The Theosophical Publishing House, Adyar, India, 1927. Thirteenth Reprint, 1996, p. 78.

A new phase begins. A grinder, no longer two parts but one solid, round mass made of light and with a handle, starts rotating over me and I get the feeling of expansion. The blockage on the right side of the chest is still there.

18 December 1996

I see a big, solid man made of silver coins, sitting cross-legged. He puts his hands up to his mouth and I see coins dropping into it like a vending machine. Then, he stretches his right palm outwards to let the silver coins fall from it.

> R. A.: This is a very singular image and this Coin-Man is not a common feature of mythical imagination – which is surprising, considering the number of phrases in all languages which are just variants of "He's made of money." From a slightly obscure Indian myth I judge that this figure is *Kubera,* the Pan-Indian god of wealth. It seems to be a highly symbolic episode. True wealth in the Indian context is Learning, which was always transmitted orally, through the Word. The stream of coins flowing from the palm is a staple of Indian myth painting to this day, and symbolises the granting of spiritual blessings or boons.

21-25 December 1996

I attended, for the first time, a four-day meditation retreat in Mahabaleshwar, for all the Mumbai students of *Brahma Vidya*. The whole experience was beautiful and exhilarating. I begin a different vibratory phase of experience, which *Guruji* calls an experience in expansion! The body becomes as light as a feather, or maybe even lighter. Actually, to describe it exactly, if I say that the body is made of air, that is what it is!

23 December 1996 (Mahabaleshwar)

The meditation was magnificent. Was it initiation or worship of the Self? In place of *Guruji* there is a *Shivalinga* moving in a circle. It comes towards me and I absorb it within me. Then, I assume that it is *Guruji* who performs the worship of me as the *Shivalinga,* first by pouring milk over my head and then water. It was all done with great love. Then, I perform the same for myself but the gentleness and the smooth movement of *Guruji* performing the same action earlier is missing to some extent and I am aware of it.

"After you become Kaula, abhisheka (ritual initiatory bath) is performed on you to make you Maha Kaula. But, mind you, you become eligible for abhisheka only when you surrender yourself completely to your guru. Only when you are completely empty can you be filled with shakti. The liquid used for abhisheka is first charged with mantric energy, so this abhisheka is a kind of Shaktipat Diksha, initiation by transfer of shakti, and it permanently alters your personality."

– *Svoboda, op. cit., p. 81.*

24 December 1996 (Mahabaleshwar)

He, who is both *Shiva* and the *Guru,* is the space in which I move, live, and have my being.

I can see *Guruji* only as Consciousness. I see him as a stretch of white sheet with a rectangle in the centre. After paying my respects I move out, leaving *Guruji* in deep meditation. Earlier, I saw the *Guru* under the canopy of Universal Consciousness, indicating to me its manifestation on the physical plane for my spiritual growth and evolution (Volume II - 12th March, 1996), and I now see him as part of the Universal Consciousness without a physical body. He representing consciousness at rest and I as consciousness in motion.

DEATH

We fear death because we are identified with the body – knowing only that this body is "I" and when this dies; it is the end of "I." This fear and the fear of the unknown makes it extremely traumatic and painful. No amount of resistance can avert the inevitable. On the contrary, it becomes a struggle. The issues related to "I Am the Doer," issues related to family, friends, relationships, disappointments, resentments, and insecurities all get together and make it a very difficult transition from one world to the other. The issues, if not resolved and dissolved during one's lifetime, become solidified and settle down in different parts of the body as energy blocks or clogged energy.

These blocks, coupled with fear and resistance to let go, cause a great deal of hindrance at the time of death. The *Prana* or energy has to move out. It has no choice but to break any form of resistance in its path, which is very painful to absorb and for the family members to watch.

The trauma of this resistance can be understood if we can identify the shift of energy in the earth's core; what power is generated for it to break through solid mass. It is the same powerful energy that is moving out of the human body and it has to destroy any resistance that comes in its path in the form of emotional, mental or physical blocks.

Just as when we are stressed and loaded with worry, we toss and turn all night and do not let sleep come near us, creating blocks of stored data. If we have resolved our problems, we look forward to a good night's restful sleep. This is also because we know that though in deep sleep "I Am not," in the waking state "I Am." I will sleep in the night and in the morning I will get up. With the same confidence we have to understand that the same principle is followed at death. We are going into deep sleep and, after a period of rest, will rise again.

The way to negate this fearful and traumatic experience is to live and die consciously.

We know that *Tattva* (element) is the substance out of which the universe is formed.

There are five *Tattvas*:

(1) *Akasha* : 'The all-pervading *Tattva*', the most refined and tenuous of the elements; directs the sense of hearing.
(2) *Vayu* : The element of air; directs the sense of touch.
(3) *Tejas* : The element of fire; directs the sense of sight.
(4) *Apas* : The element of water; directs the sense of taste.
(5) *Prithvi* : The element of earth; directs the sense of smell.

Tattvas are manifested in gross and subtle forms. Every gross form has its subtle counterpart. Just as the universe is formed of *Tattvas*, the human body is the gross form of the five vital airs. The physical, mental, and emotional levels and every nerve current of the human body is governed by that *Tattva* which has control of it. Each *Tattva* has its positive and negative phases. If all the *Tattvas* are balanced we can lead a harmonious existence. This is an impossible task, for each thought, each act, and every effort of the will excites the *Tattvic* vibration, and its affect on the body-mind intellect depends on the intensity of the same. A diseased body is the result of disturbed *Tattvic* law. As this realisation dawns, life becomes simpler and we move towards harmony within and without.

So, what happens at death?

If one has understood the law of nature and the *Tattvas,* depending how consciously one has lived, and if one has the knowledge and understanding of the principle, "I Am That," the *Prana* will move out accordingly.

"The vital breath is leaving the body, the 'I Amness' receding, but the 'I Amness' is going to the Absolute. That is the greatest moment, the greatest moment of immortality. The 'I Amness' was there, that movement was there, and I observe, it is extinguished. The ignorant one will get very frightened at the moment of death – he is struggling – but for the jnani, it is the happiest moment."

– Dunn, Jean – 'Prior to Consciousness – Talks with Sri Nisargadatta Maharaj'. Chetana Pvt. Ltd., Mumbai, India. First Indian Edition, 1998, p. 23.

If one is relaxed in the moment of death, having understood the working of existence, the subtle elements will start dispersing and dissolving in their universal whole and the *Prana* will move out to merge with the Source, waiting for the next movement in consciousness. I view this experience of 'Death' as the 'Birth' of a soul. It's an ongoing cycle of birth and birth – from the subtle to the gross and from the gross to the subtle. "There is no death, there is no death, there is no death. Death is not the law of life; law of creation is the law of life."

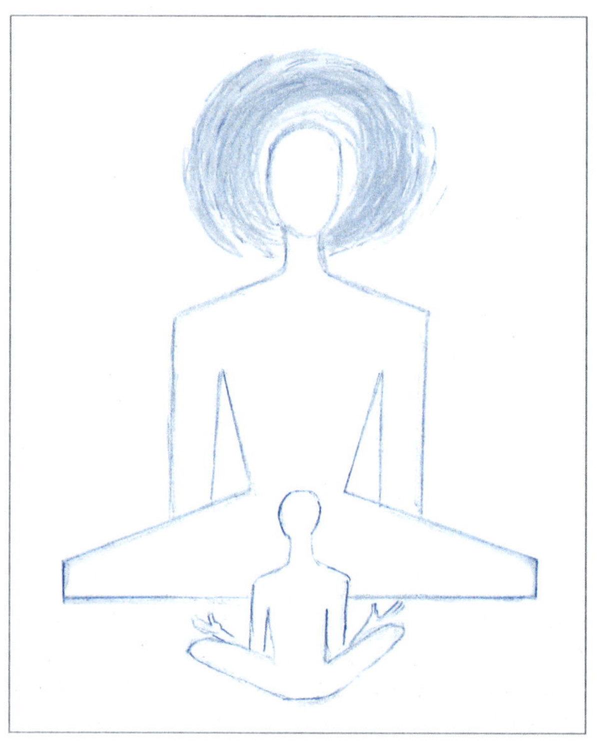

Chapter Two

THE TEACHER AND THE TAUGHT

My progress is still constantly monitored; I am still assisted to help the flow of energy. This has been conducted mainly by applying pressure on the toes or certain areas of the feet. This acupressure has been going on for some months now. Whenever applied, I feel a smoother flow of energy. The pressure gives direction to the energy. Also, the emphasis seems to be in the chest region. Here, the pressure comes in the form of a shock, given by a sudden thrust; the body jerks like the patients who are given electric shock treatment.

I also notice that I am no longer seeing the 'yellow, orange, or gold light', which emanates from within the body, but the emphasis is now on 'white light'. This light, when it comes in a flash, is blinding and when I am bathed in this light, it is totally soothing, giving a profound sense of being nurtured and cherished. There are no words to describe the experience of the Source. I can only try with my limited vocabulary and expression, and that too does not really seem to do justice.

1 January 1997

I see myself climbing up the Axis of the Earth. The Axis has protrusions like that of the vertebrae of the spine. The realisation dawns that the human spine is the extension of the Axis or the Earth spine, thus, serving as a conduit between the Sun energy and the Earth energy.

R. A.: The axis being referred to here is of course the *Axis Mundi,* the centre of the universe. In the Hindu tradition it is called the *Yupa Stambha,* the Cosmic Pillar that the universe is supported by as well as rotates around. A Hindu temple, when properly designed, makes of every man a *Yupa Stambha* when he is correctly aligned before the deity. As Santosh has correctly deduced, the human spine is regarded as the *Yupa Stambha.* In fact, *Tantra* explicitly calls the spinal column the *Meru Danda. Meru* is the cosmic mountain at the centre of the universe and *Danda* is the royal staff of authority as well as the power of punishing evil. Complete conscious awareness of the spine results in the Ultimate Centring. This is always accompanied by alterations in breath patterns and conscious states. In Iconography, realised souls (like the Buddha or Surya) are always depicted as standing bolt upright as though they have been frameworked in steel. They have the consciousness of the *Meru Danda* within them. Being Centred at the very immovable heart of the universe, they therefore speak with authority (*danda*). Man is thus the centre of the universe in a spiritual sense. The *Kundalini* twines itself around or through this *Yupa Stambha.* The shape of her pillar reminds us of the temple flag posts found in many parts of India, and they too are stand-ins for the *Yupa Stambha.* Until the *Kundalini* climbs the *Meru Danda* fully and reaches the Crown *chakra* however, the experience of having the *Meru Danda* within is more theoretical than a reality.

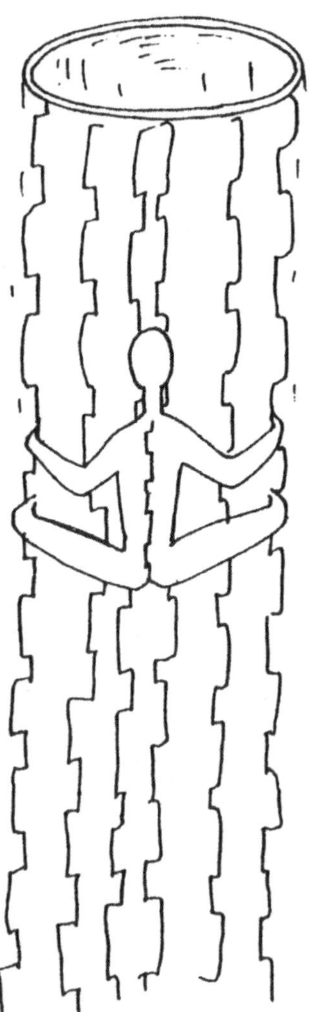

4 January 1997

Group meditation at the Guru's residence: I start to feel the energy rise very purposefully in a spiral form, at the same time creating a sinking sensation in the heart, as if the life force is being pulled out. I ignore that and let the energy proceed upwards, simultaneously experiencing a sense of dispersing and getting scattered all over in tiny particles; the only thing intact being the consciousness. The whole procedure is quite fast and does not give me time to think. I stay scattered and it is a wonderful feeling. Consciousness registers the *Guru's Omkara* (the call to come out of meditation) but takes its own time to gather itself from its dispersed state. Consciousness also registers that after a bit of silence *Guruji* starts a normal course of conversation, thus giving me my space and enabling me to gather myself and make a gradual descent. I am also aware that I have to take it easy and get completely integrated.

It is a breathtaking experience.

One young aspirant who went through the above experience and who literally forced herself out of meditation on hearing the *Omkara,* experienced a great sense of disorientation and nausea which lasted for a couple of days. Having gone through my experience, I was able to understand where she had gone wrong to her great discomfort. I advised her that henceforth when she went through the experience of dispersing, she should not try to rush out of that state, but allow the experience to take its natural course and time and let a gradual descent happen. Only then there is completion and a feeling of wholeness.

Now, at times I can feel my whole body vibrating and my movement from one vibratory level to another is smoother. The above experience started the process of expansion in me.

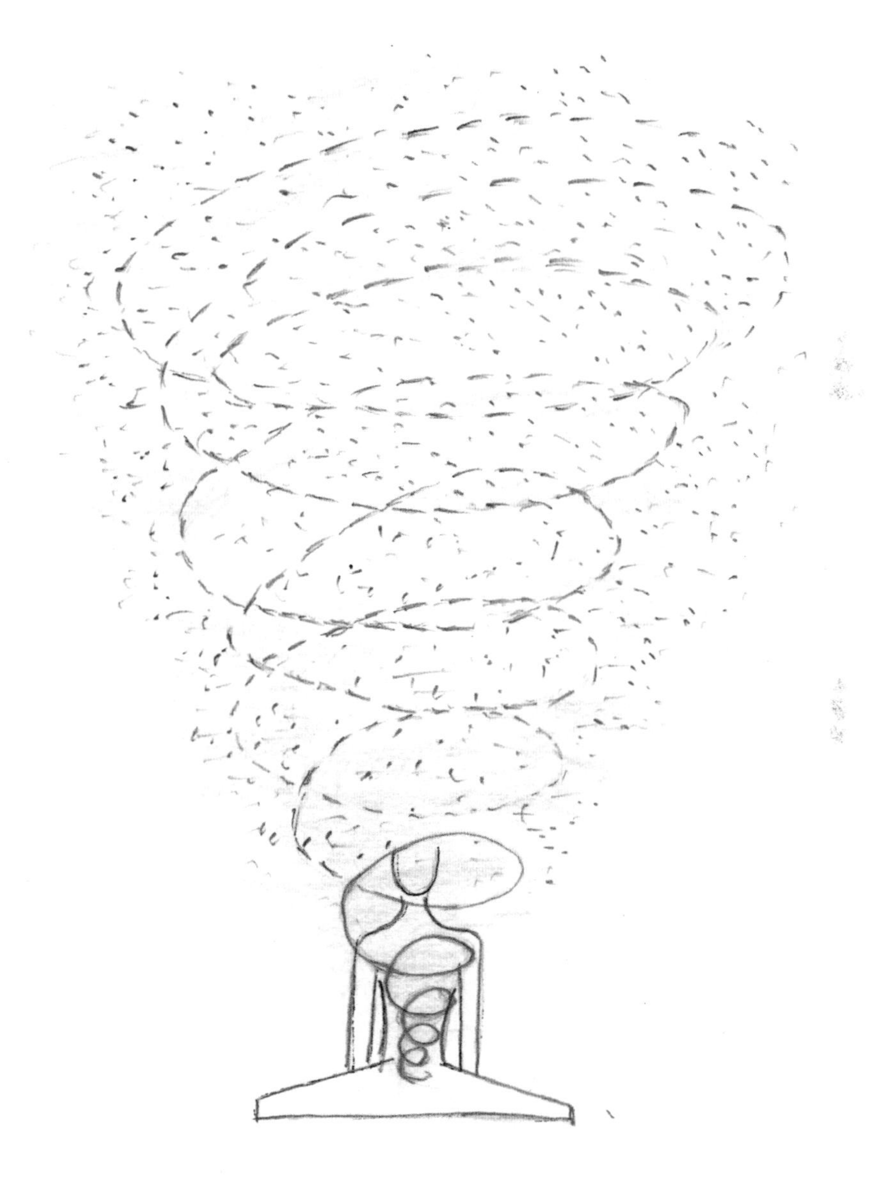

7 January 1997

I am neither body nor the mind.

Slight apprehension –

While I am in a state of flux, I cannot locate my mind or body till I change back from subtle vibration to a denser vibration.

As I am identified with Cosmic Consciousness, a wrapped-up, sick, newborn baby is placed in my arms.

It is fascinating to know that every thought, word and action is actually arising and merging in the One Source Consciousness. If I live in constant awareness, I realise that even in fragmentation, my experience is in 'Wholeness'. I am reminded of hot springs where the 'Whole' is constantly bubbling, rising and merging – rising and merging.

10 January 1997

During meditation, my face appears larger-than-life, and a long needle traces its way along the jaw line and, then, along the cheeks. There is light and more light. A left hand is placed on the right side of my chest, in line with the armpit. The top of the hand is tapped with the right hand. This is the area where I feel the blockage. The blockage does not clear immediately, but does so in due course.

14 January 1997

The body is absorbing pink – the *chakra* that is working is the *Manipur*.

I see myself standing on a burnished rocky surface, watching a flowing river of fire. One day, I was watching the Discovery Channel on television and much to my awe and surprise, the underground flow of the lava that was being shown was the one I had been standing on. My consciousness had gone down into the core of the earth. Even though I was standing on the red-hot surface, there was no sense of burning.

25 January 1997

There is a knocking with a chisel and hammer going on in my chest.

The doors open wide in the chest, indicating that my *Anahat chakra* (Heart *chakra*) is fully operative.

28 January 1997

Prana moves out of the point below the left breast and, after expansion, comes as a laser beam and starts entering the right side of the chest.

29 January 1997

A cord with a knot is pulled out of the chest and it snaps at the knotted point.

After all the activity going on in the chest, there is a tremendous feeling of lightness and free flow of energy.

5 February 1997

Morning meditation: The body gets light. It starts moving from mid-section, spreading into four distinct directions.

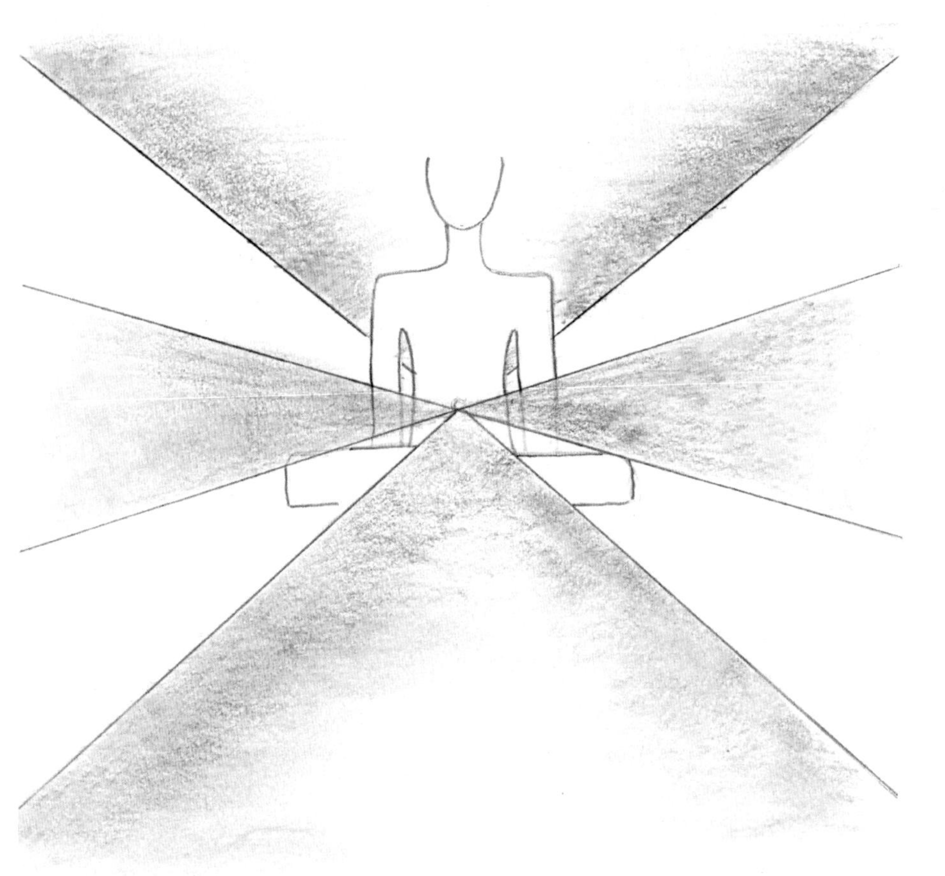

5 February 1997

Then, I find that I start expanding upwards until I feel that I will probably go out of the roof.

In spite of the great expansion and growing to an unimaginable size, I was surprised to note that there was no heaviness to the body. On the contrary, there was a feeling of extreme lightness. I had no weight. During the experience I did not realise that it was the etheric body that had expanded. When I joined the course, I did not know that anything like the etheric body or any other body than the gross body existed.

After becoming fully familiar with the feeling of expansion, I started to move towards the powerful experience of the White Light, whether it was descending or ascending.

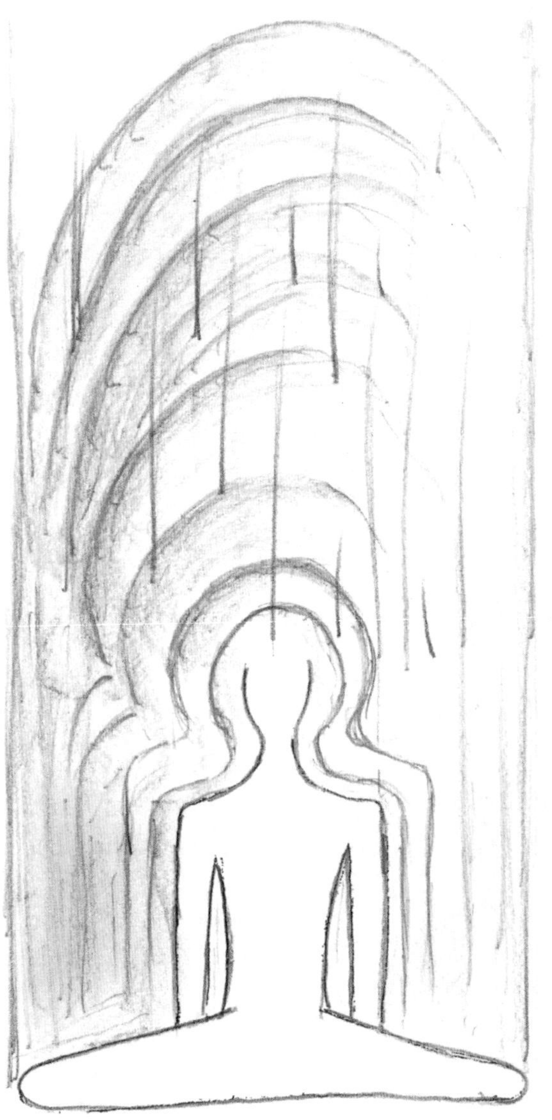

11 February 1997

During meditation, the chest is like a sea of gold with a golden boat heaving in it.

I see my body as a battleground with hordes of elephants led by a royal elephant running in full force, as if for attack. There are horses with warriors dashing on the battlefield – my body.

A golden force settles in my chest.

14 February 1997

Energy, as a fiery thread throwing sparks of joyous current, traces its course upwards along the spine, through the *Sushumna nadi.*

"Kundalini has been described as vidyut lata, the 'lightning creeper'. Think of how a creeping vine clings to a tree; and then think of that vine as a lightning stroke, a bolt of billions of volts of energy which would splinter or incinerate any ordinary tree, or bush."

– Svoboda, op. cit., p. 61.

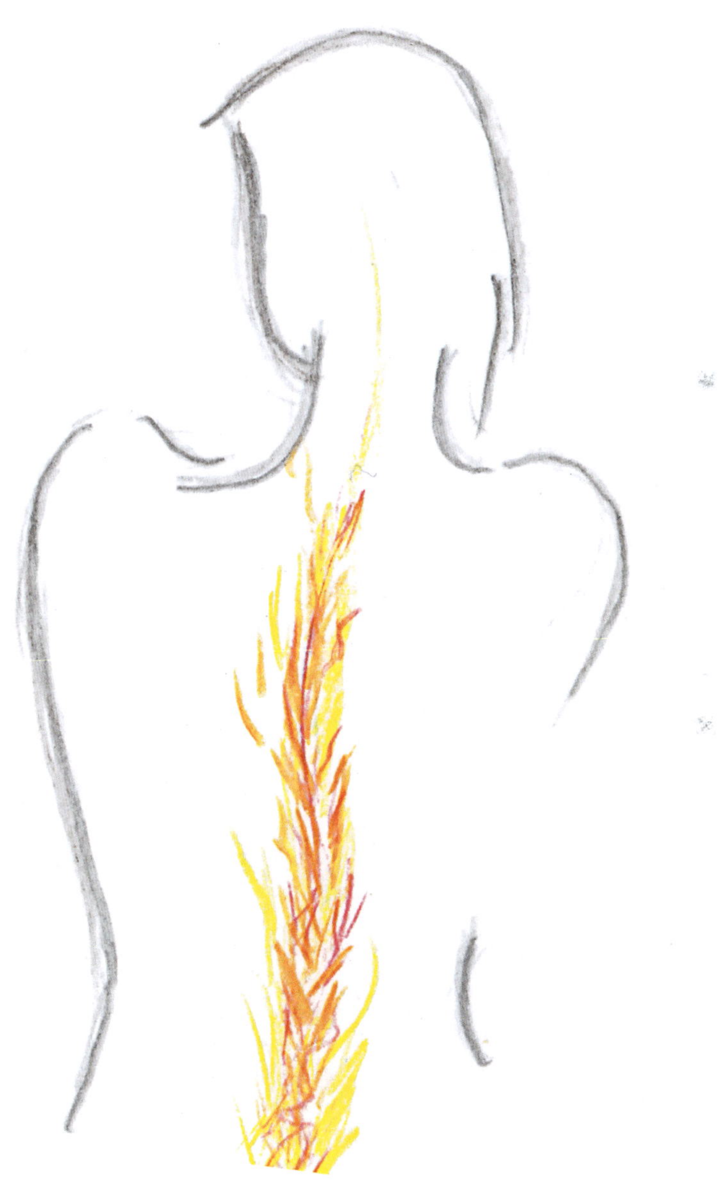

25 February 1997

Group meditation at the Guru's residence: A shape like a dish antenna appears over the head. The antenna starts moving in different directions like a radar. This is probably the vibration of the *Sahasrar* giving the particular shape.

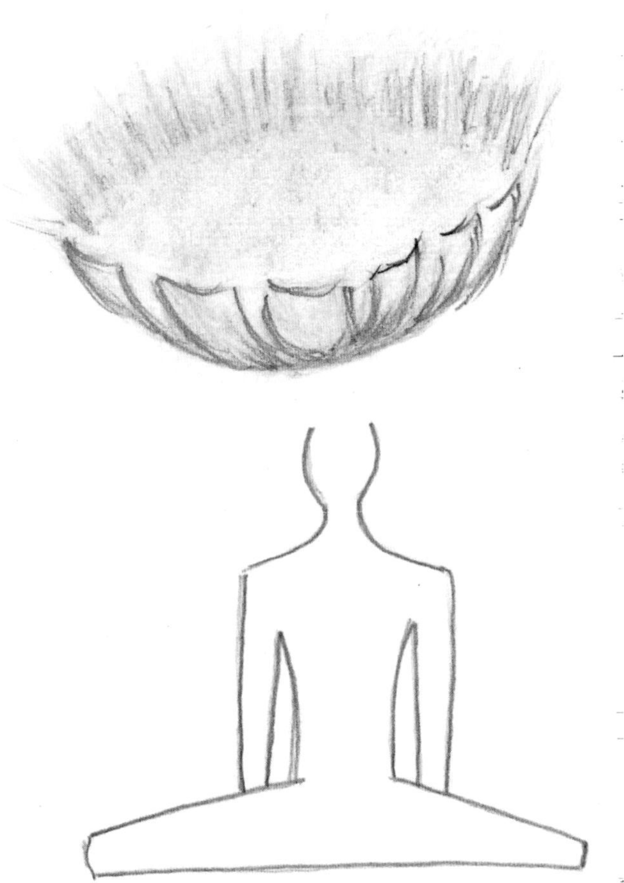

27 February 1997

The body starts merging with the cosmic energy till there is no body left except a bright star.

27 February 1997

Afternoon: I am looking at a blood report and hear a voice saying there is a weakness in the body. I say, "take care of it then." I see myself standing over me and my complexion is ash blue in colour. I watch myself and then my blue self slowly disappears into my Self.

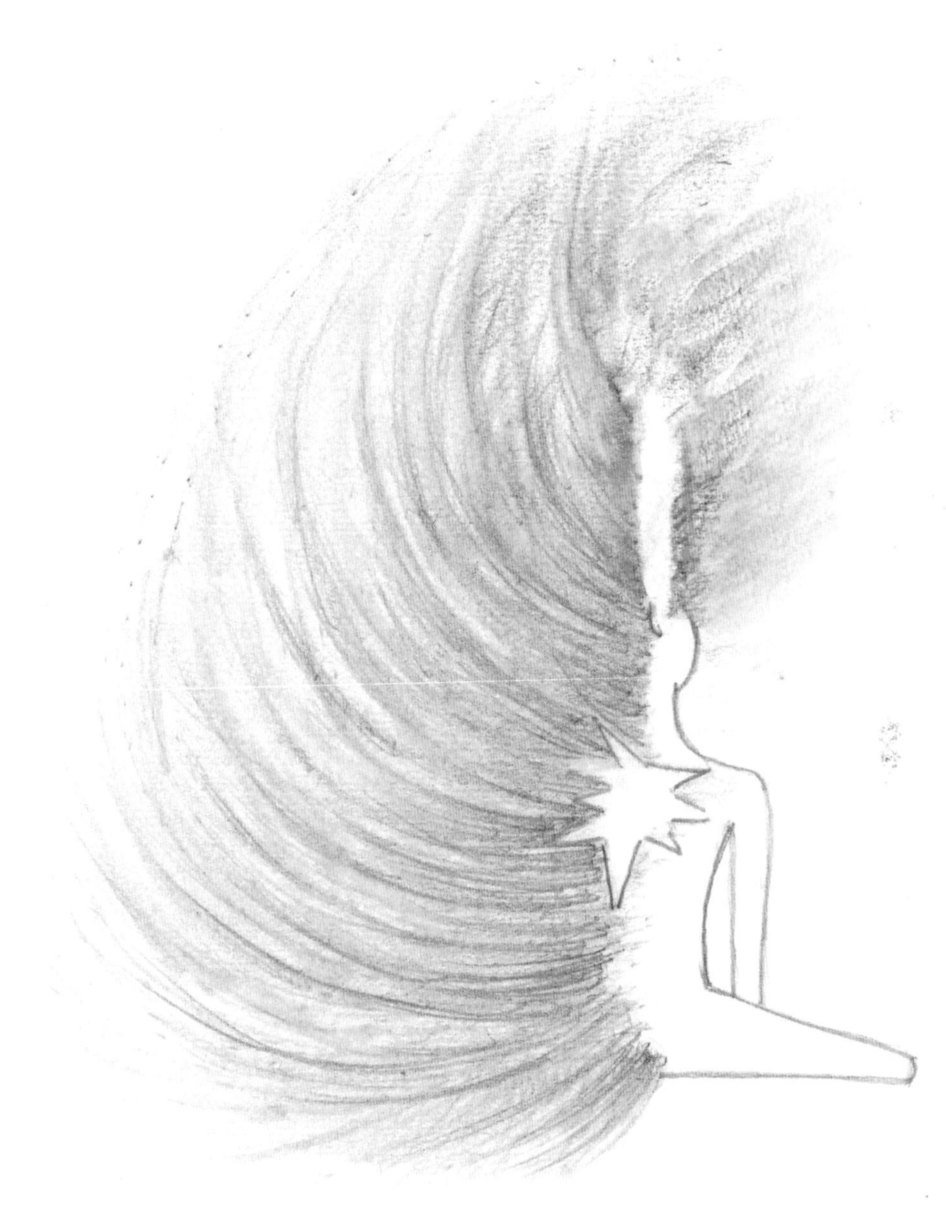

28 February 1997

I keep moving upwards till I am just a white circle of vacuum in space with an energy field moving around me. *Guruji* says that this is the region of *'Om'*.

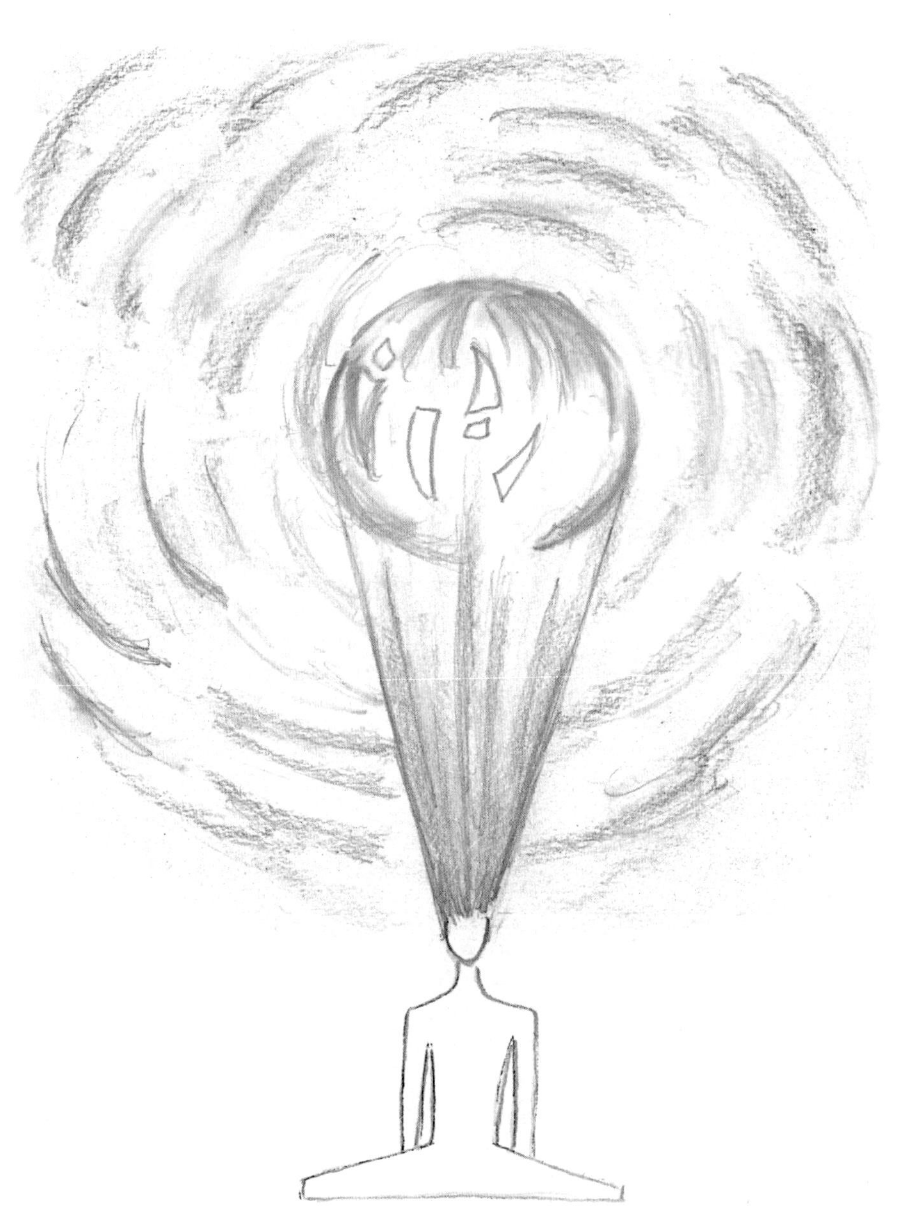

4 March 1997

4:30 am: The chest feels as if it were a cement block. The energy has settled there.

8 am: The right side of the body seems to get heavy and begins stretching towards the right and then up. The feeling is as if a magnet is pulling the body. I hear the clear sound of a flute playing, sometimes close and sometimes at a distance.

12 March 1997
(Moving into the Dimension of White Light)

I am meditating, but I find myself in the void. I seem to be caught in some cosmic confusion with what seems to me like a volley of atoms flying around me. This seems to have formed a pattern till I inform *Guruji* about it. After that, the pattern stops. I feel that my body atoms were being rearranged so that it would be receptive to the experience that was to follow.

After this, a new phase starts for me where I have the experience of white light. There is no more yellow or golden light. There are no more colours, only white light and more white light.

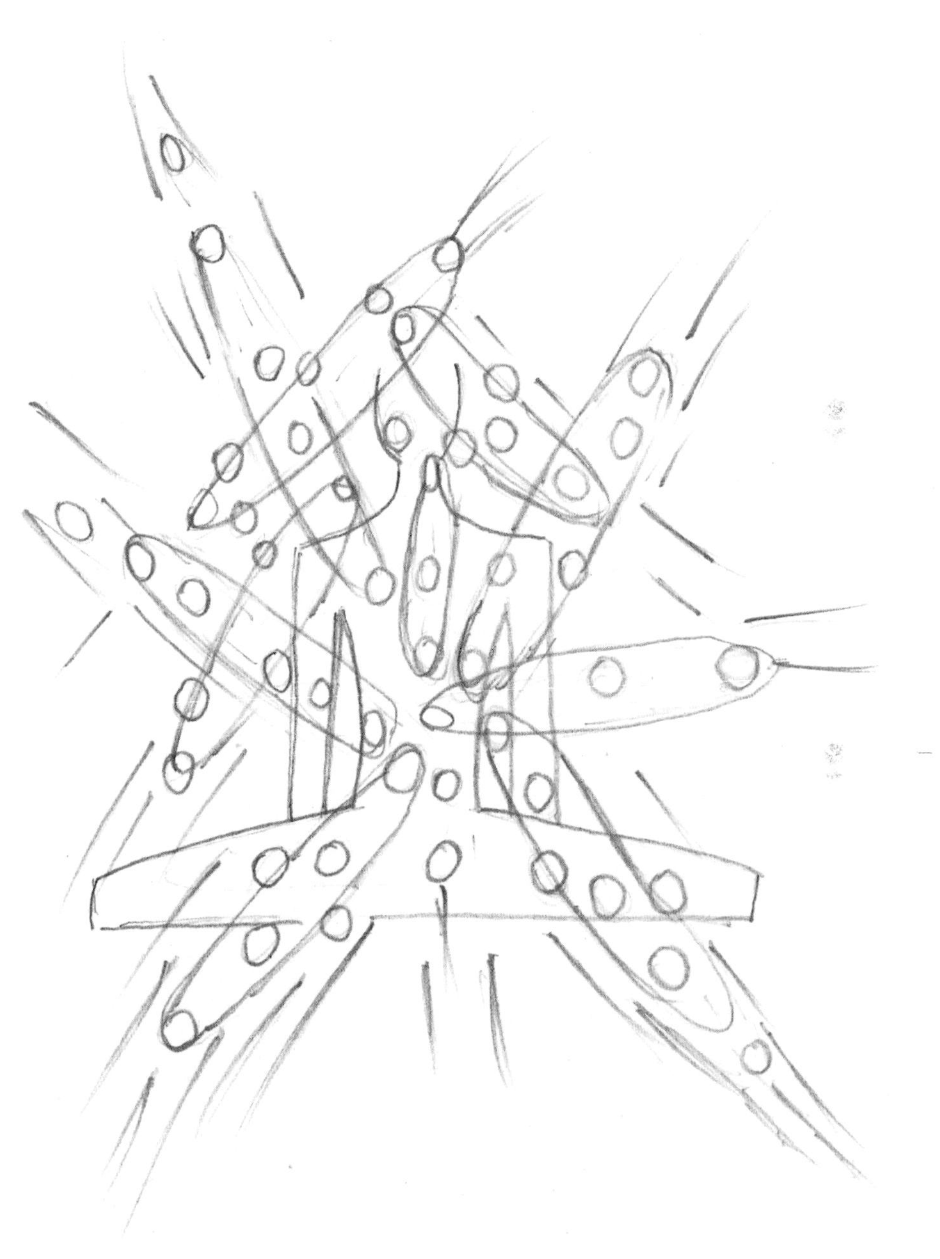

12 March 1997

Morning meditation: I feel and see white light coming towards me from all directions. It is like a wall of light. It stops at about two feet from me, surrounding me from all directions. I can sense the solidity of it.

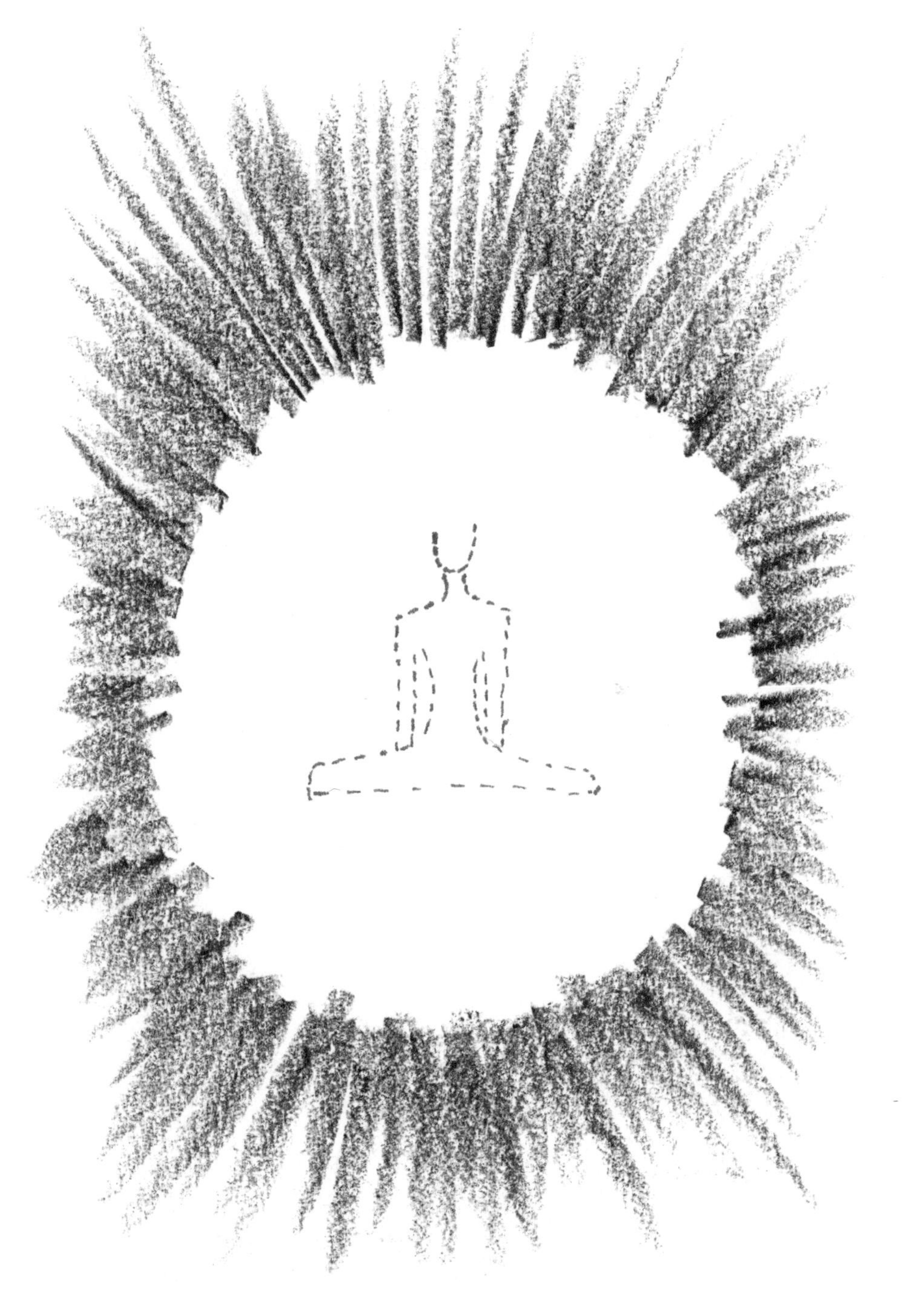

12 March 1997

The white light settles in the right side of my chest and starts to radiate outwards in all directions.

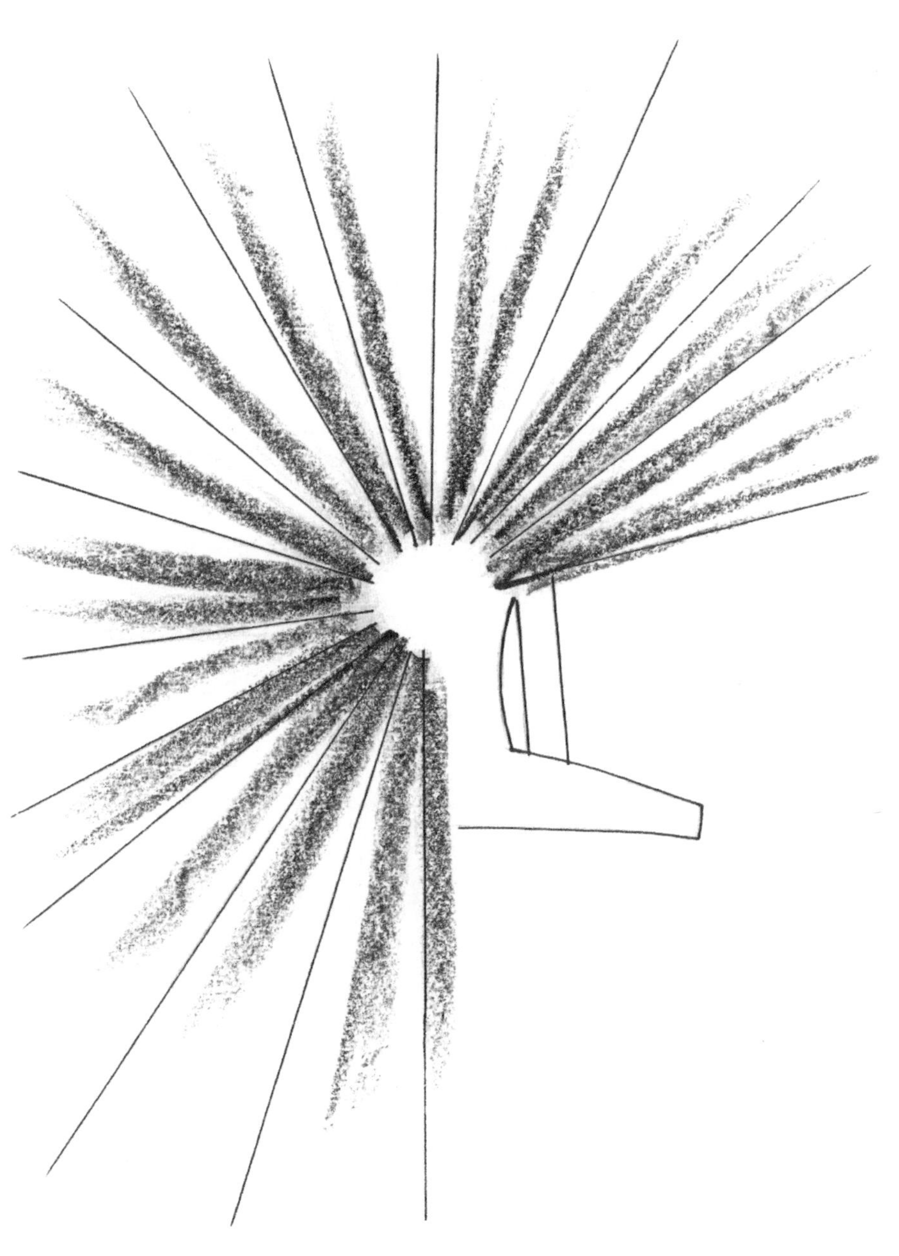

13 March 1997

Two people remove my body from a grave and dump it on the ground. I am a black stretch of beach that goes on pushing at the Black Sea. Then, I start flowing towards my body till I become a tunnel that starts like a black worm. There are tongues of flames going through the tunnel. I see a black form, with flames flying from it, coming towards my body. The form is coming in some sort of chariot. Then, I see a stretch of glossy, creamish, closely knitted, smooth pebbles. I, as in Consciousness, am hovering in the brain. On the right side of the brain, spinning activity is going on over me. I am in the twilight zone, and a dark, reddish glow starts flowing into me.

R. A.: The black form with flames emerging from a tunnel is symbolic of the birth of consciousness. It is normally experienced as the Sun-Chariot in myth as nothing could be a better metaphor for consciousness emergent from the darkness of unawareness. It is interesting that Helios, the spiritual sun of Greek myth as opposed to Apollo – the visible sun, is a black sun. It is experienced as black because directly gazing into the Light of Consciousness blinds you. Santosh distinctly says she experiences herself as Consciousness. The peculiar 'pebbles' look very much like the knit bones of the skull, seen as they would be if laid out flat!

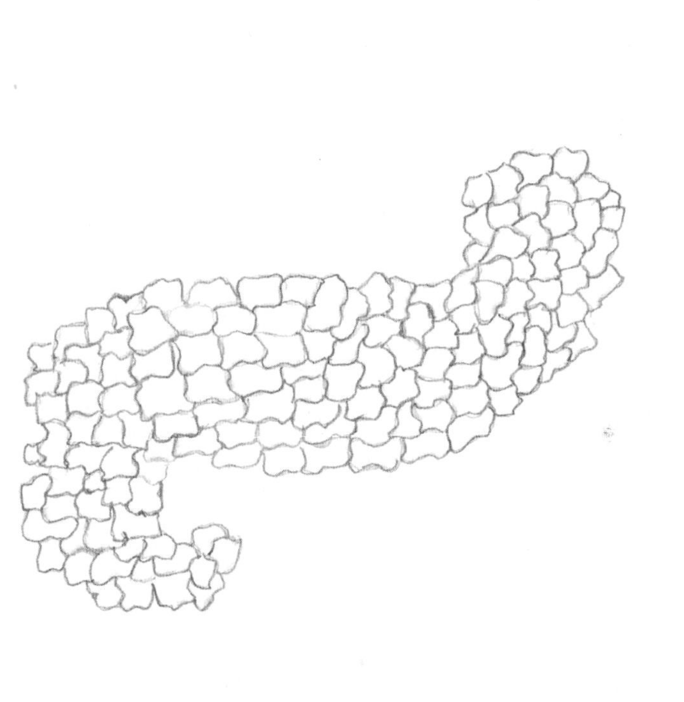

18 March 1997

Morning meditation: I see *Guruji* and myself sitting for meditation. I see *Guruji's* form get out of his body, my form get out of my body. Both walk towards each other and merge.

"Shiva is within Shakti and Shakti is within Shiva. When Shakti is unmanifest, Shiva is absolute and alone. When Shakti is in a state of becoming, Shiva appears like the creator." (Mokashi-Punekar, p. 43-44, 51-52, 57)

Govindan, Marshall – 'Babaji and the 18 Siddha Kriya Yoga Tradition'. Babaji's Kriya Yoga Order of Acharyas Trust, Malleswaram West, Bangalore, India, 2003. p. 46.

I sought Thee in the timeless halls of space
I sought Thee in the spaceless halls of time
But found that time and space do not exist.
I wondered 'Who am I?' and 'Who art Thou?'
And then I found Thee. Thou in me and I in Thee.
'Twas then I knew that I do not exist.
For I am nothing; yet am everything
For evermore... and so we cannot die.

– Goslin, Robert – Synchronicity Inner Network #714.

R. A.: Every once in a while, the *Kundalini* experiences remind Santosh of her identification with the *Guru*. This is a vital safeguard on this path and not just a repetitive visual tic as it were. Each time it occurs is a distinct and fresh reminder valuable in itself, not as a habit of thought or as an affirmation. The relationship with the *Guru* transcends all other experience and it would be catastrophic to lose sight of it.

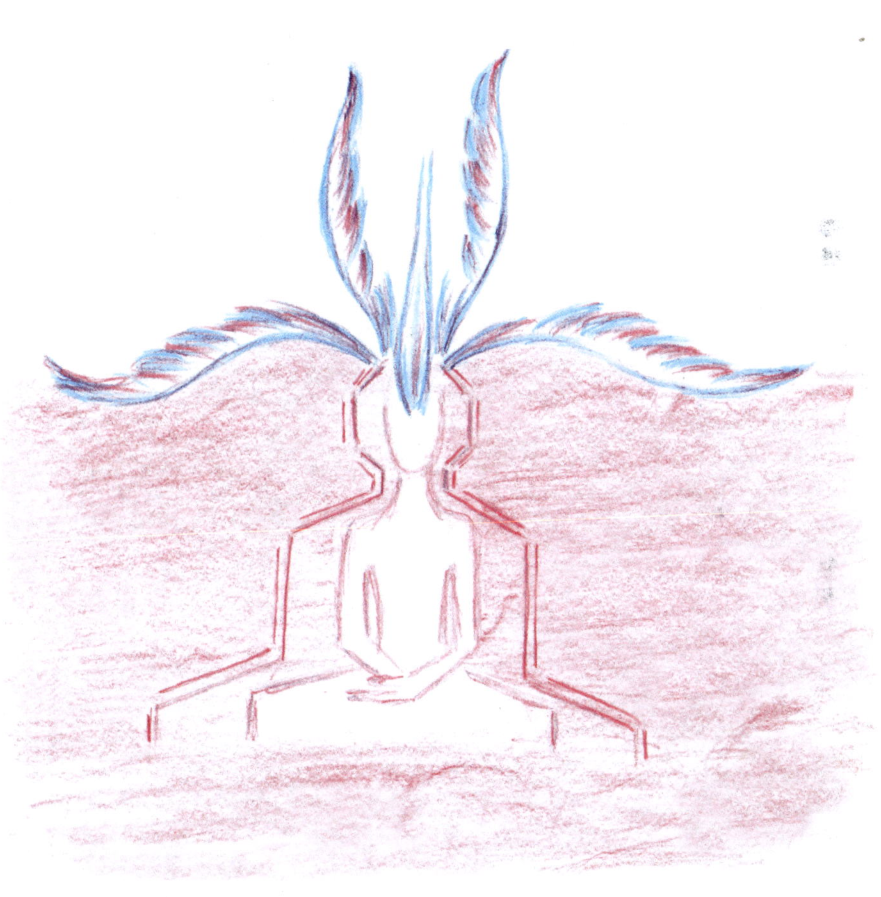

18 March 1997

My progress is still being monitored from another realm. Invisible hands gently place a strap around my neck and a plug in my hand. A large gadget is placed on the right side of my head and it is recording the brain activity.

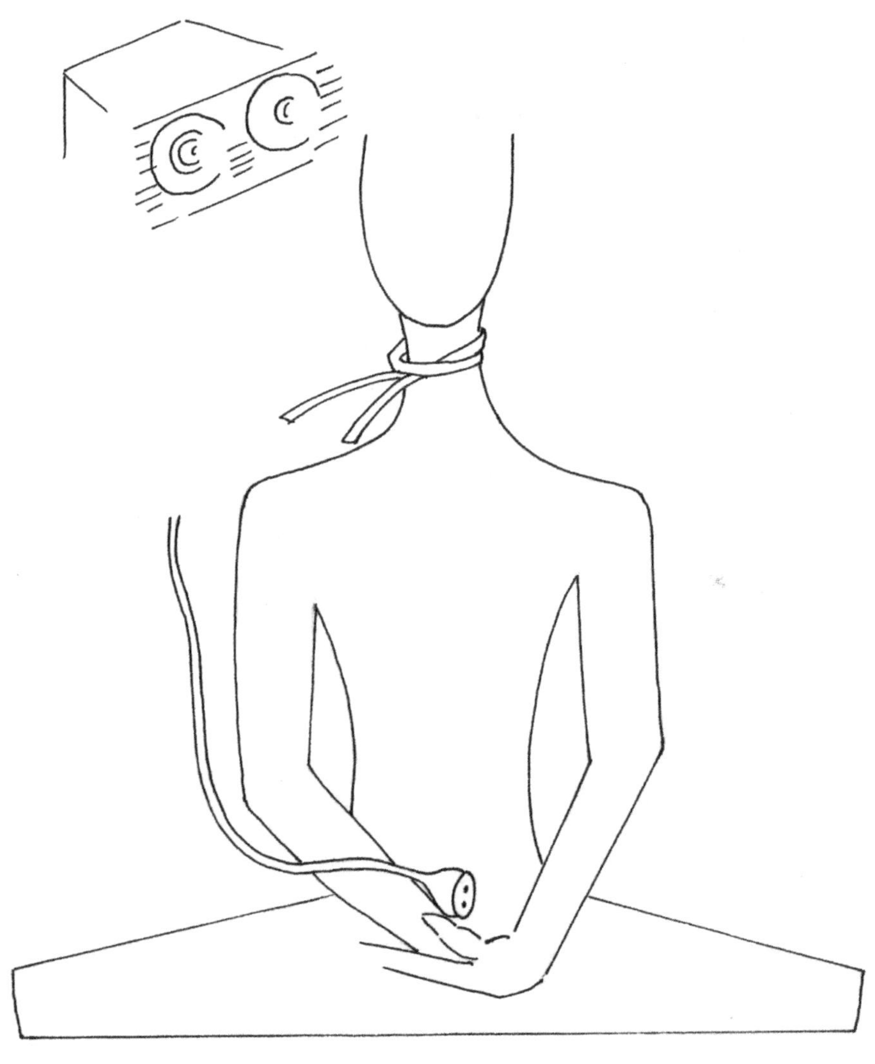

20 March 1997

I see figures in white. I see a woman's face very close to me. Her head is covered. She is looking at me. I become aware and acknowledge her look. She has elongated eyes, more like Oriental features. A man dressed in white walks towards me, gets down on one knee. Awareness is at chest level.

I am guided into a narrow room with high walls and when I am brought out, I am made of white light.

10 April 1997

Today was different. There was constant rhythmic ticking somewhere between the forehead and the nose. For the meditation, only the left nostril functioned. Got up feeling very light.

13 April 1997

12:30 am: In a dream, I see myself sitting with the *Guru* in a group meditation. At one stage, *Guruji* takes my hand in his hand. I give the *Omkara.* There are people though I don't see them. Then, *Guruji* helps me get up and guides me out and tells the boys that I am to be taken safely home. Somebody asks, "Who else will be in the bus?" *Guruji* says, "Her father." The father is the same man as the one when I was a farmer boy, but he is sitting in front and his back is towards me. At one stage, I stand on the seat to close the air vent. It turns into a beam. A tea boy wants to give me a mug of tea, but he wants me to hold it in a particular fashion – I don't take it, because he will not let me look into the cup. I wake up. When I narrated the dream to *Guruji,* he said that I should have taken the cup as offered. I missed a gift!

19 April 1997
(Meeting with Papaji of Swami Narayan Sect.)

'Yogi Divine Society' is part of the Swami Narayan group. I was led to this society through a book *Essence of Tantra*. Here I came in contact with Bharat bhai, Vashi bhai, Raju bhai, Kanti bhai and others. The sense of belonging with the group was complete. There was a sense of oneness of spirit without a distinction of gender.

Raju bhai of Yogi Divine Society called me and invited me to meet Papaji who had come from Gujarat and was on his way to London the same night. I took my manuscript and met Raju bhai below their ashram at Navjeevan Society, Tardeo. As we sat in the black Sumo an old man joined us, getting in the front seat. The driver's seat was occupied by a young aspirant who was unfamiliar with a Sumo and Mumbai's roads. Bharat bhai shouted from the fourth floor: "Drive carefully." We settled in for a long bumpy drive to Kandivili. I was looking around the car to check if there was an air conditioner and was told that it was not functioning. As we reached the ashram the lights went off and I was made to wait in a room where there were lady *sadhvis*. When the lights came on I saw a big group of devotees crowding in a room where an elderly gentleman dressed in crisp white was reclining in a chair with his feet resting, stretched out on a stool. There were others waiting out for their turn to be in the energy field of the Master. As the lights came on one of the lady *sadhvis* was insisting that I go in, not realising that there was no space to manoeuvre myself in that packed place. She made some gesture and the room started to clear till there was no one left. I walked in peacefully, put my manuscript on a chair, and knelt at the feet of Papaji, asking to sit with him for meditation. After meditation, I caught hold of his feet and placed my forehead on them; he invited me to sit beside him and narrate my experience. I went on in my enthusiastic manner, enjoying every moment and basking in the love that was shining in Papaji's eyes. The crowd outside started getting restless and it was announced that Papaji had to prepare for his flight.

19 April 1997 (Contd.)

I was taken to the dining area and given some refreshments. Everyone gathered outside to bid farewell to Papaji. I stood in a corner not wanting to intrude on the congregation's space. I was a total stranger to them. Papaji's car came. He saw me standing. He stretched out his left hand, palm up. I went forward and placed my hand in his.

This gesture of Papaji left me completely awe struck and wonder struck. It seemed that in that one moment he had taught me the meaning of 'Unconditional Love & Surrender'.

The whole trip to Kandivili was very familiar till I realised that it was following the same pattern and sequence played out in my dream; the black Sumo representing the bus, the old man in the front seat I recognised as my father from a past life as a farmer. Bharat bhai shouting from above to drive carefully and one young man escorting me while the other was to drive. The woman who was to join us dropped out at the last minute. It was my *Guru* who sent me out to meet this great sage; who with his single gesture transformed a part of me.

30 April 1997

I am standing in my chest, with a *puja thali* in my hand. A figure in *dhoti,* sleeveless jacket, and a turban, bows down deep in front of me – I sprinkle something (maybe rice and *kumkum*) on his head and bless him. As soon as awareness occurs, a sheet of light goes through my body.

1 May 1997

I feel pain and pressure in the right foot above the toes, followed by free flow of energy.

> R. A.: For quite some time now Santosh had been reporting pain and other peculiar sensations in the feet. The feet are the repository of the energy of Grace, and the problems and discomfort she was having has to do with the organism adjusting to this influx of energy.

2 May 1997

Pain and pressure is applied in the left foot, at an angle from the ankle, followed by free flow of energy.

15 May 1997

4 am: A powerful light is falling from behind over the left shoulder. My mouth starts to open wide and stretches to the maximum and stays that way. There is total merging with the cosmos.

17 May 1997

I see myself in the cremation grounds where a funeral pyre is burning. I am a lean, young man with long hair, upper body bare. I have a round, big, black bowl in my hands. There is ash and fire in it. I'm reciting something and then lift the bowl over my head and turn it upside down and pour the ash and fire over myself. I am left with a feeling of euphoria and exhilaration.

> R. A.: This was clearly a memory of *sadhana* in the past life – the famous *Agni-Snan*, or Fire-Bath, to rather dramatically and drastically purify oneself by being laved with fire. Obviously, something very important was resolved with this memory surfacing. The feeling of joy that Santosh felt is possible only if there is some closure to an ongoing issue – in a *karmic* sense, which is free of linear notions of time. Many of these visions are signposts telling Santosh that certain practices or actions have culminated as they ought to, so there is no need to have them linger in the subconscious.

12:45 pm: There is too much energy in the body, with the result that I can't sleep. I am trying to keep myself on the ground. I realise that my body wants to lift itself up. I let go, and I'm flying with a quiet, swishing sound – I fly off somewhere. It seems just a second or two, and I find that I'm still in bed in the same posture that I left.

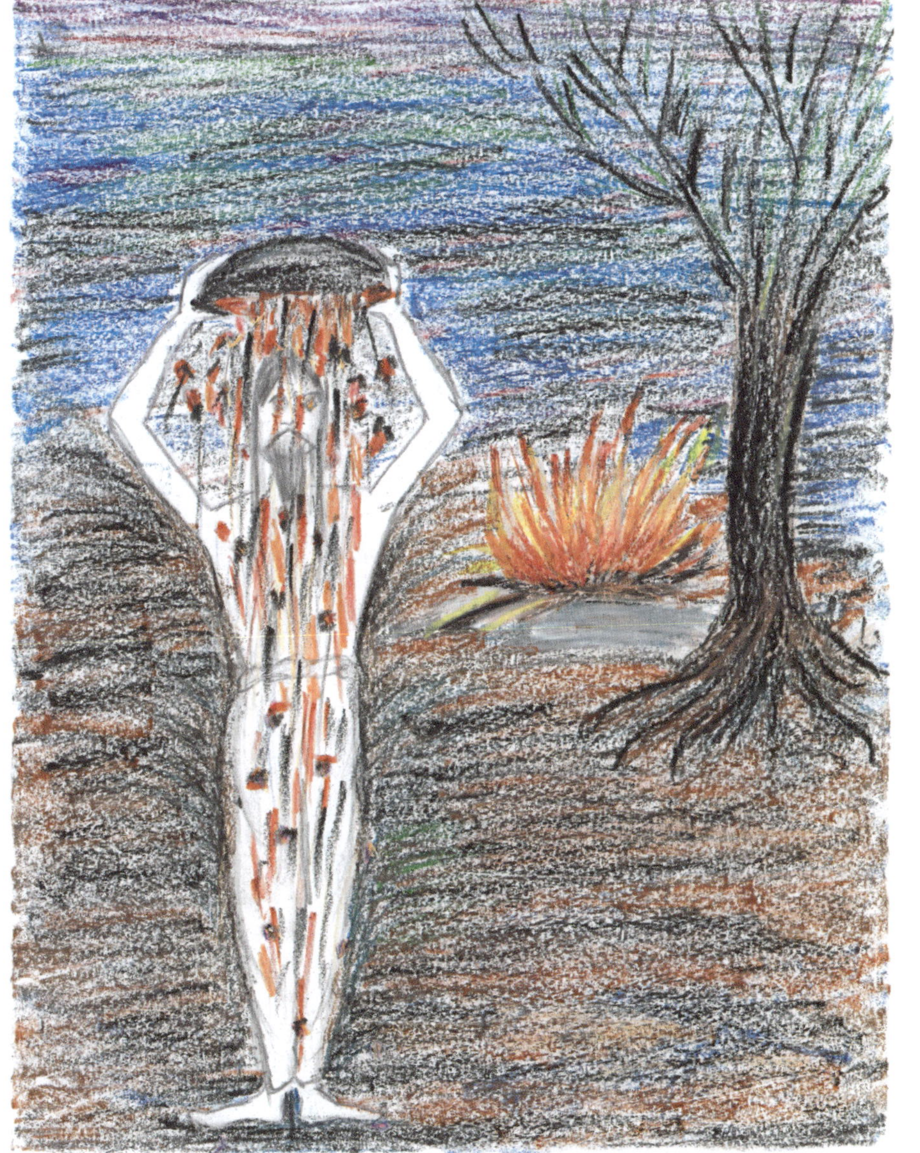

22 May 1997

I had a most powerful experience. The bed moved as if the earth had shifted. The whole body was charged with energy. With the invocation to the *Guru,* I left myself open to the energy. This probably happened because the *Muladhar chakra* suddenly became active.

3 June 1997

Today, I heard a very heavy and soft sound, first in the right ear and later in the left. The sound was heavy and resonant – more like *Bhannnn.* This is the echo of the beat of a massive drum.

16 June 1997

This evening, I see groups of men dressed in white, performing different functions. It seems like they are preparing for a *yagna*. Prominent among them is a handsome *Sardarji* wearing a colourful, decorative turban, a long coat and *churidar-pyjama*. He reminds me of a *Sikh Guru*. He is circumambulating through the crowd of people in a gliding movement.

17 June 1997

A new beginning. Dark maroon, rose-like flowers flow into the lower left side of my body, across it and then, changing their course upwards, they move out of it. From my forehead, there is a stem going up with a *chakra* rotating on it, throwing rays of silver light.

"Now this etheric double has often been called the vehicle of the human life-ether or vital force (called in Sanskrit prana), and anyone who has developed the psychic faculties can see exactly how this is so. He will see the solar life-principle almost colourless, though intensely luminous and active, which is constantly poured into the earth's atmosphere by the sun; he will see how the etheric part of his spleen in the exercise of its wonderful function absorbs this universal life, and specializes it into prana, so that it may be more readily assimilable by his body; how it then courses all over that body, running along every nerve-thread in tiny globules of lovely rosy light, causing the glow of life and health and activity to penetrate every atom of the etheric double; and how, when the rose-coloured particles have been absorbed, the superfluous life-ether finally radiates from the body in every direction as bluish white light."

– Leadbeater, C. W. – 'Dreams: What they are and how they are caused'. The Theosophical Publishing House, Adyar, India, 1898. Fifteenth Reprint, 1997, pp. 7-8.

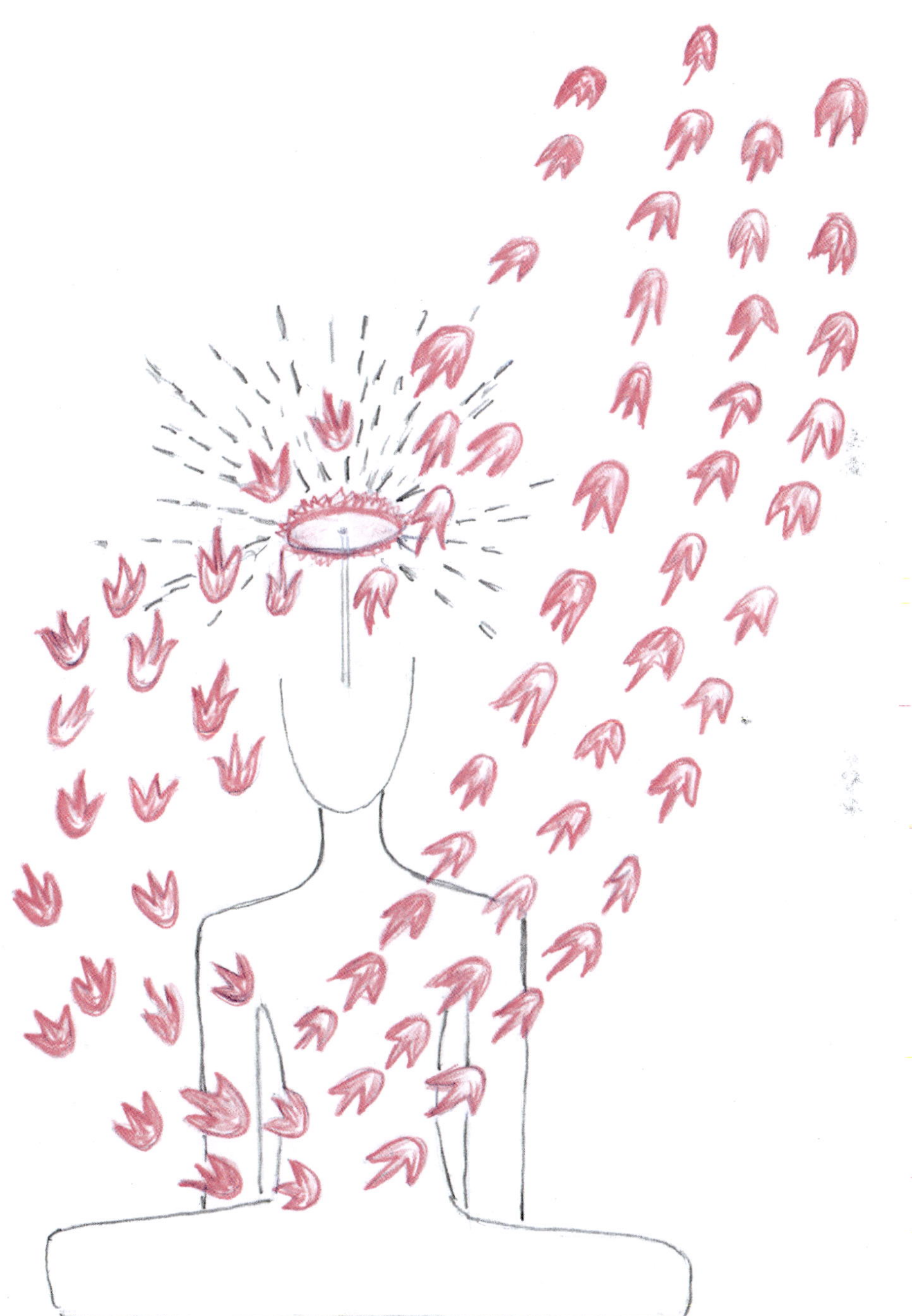

20 June 1997

There are small balls coming from space and I am trying to catch them. There are eyes watching me.

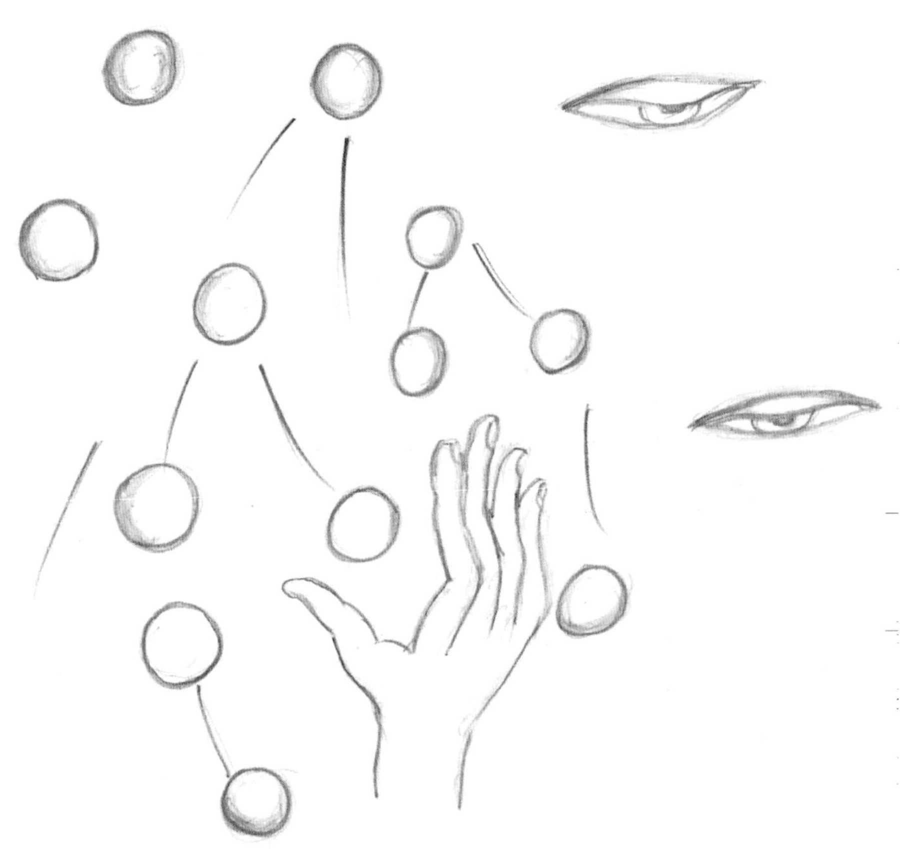

7 July 1997

During meditation, I see myself as a man of prehistoric times, on my knees, with a stick or some object in my hands, arms raised up and my face lifted to the sun, worshipping it. I am bathed in the sun's rays and I start moving into them towards the sun. The arms, raised in invocation to the sun, also raised my consciousness.

15 July 1997

My left brain was being filled with some matter.

Group meditation at the Guru's residence: I see myself as a still patch of water, and the reflections are upside down in me.

16 July 1997

While drawing the visuals, the mug with the paint-brushes caught my eye and, lo and behold, I am a mug of water with paintbrushes in it. I am fascinated by the play of consciousness. If I were to get stuck in one of these situations, what would I be termed as?! This is a very serious business and one cannot be playful about it. If one has to be playful, it has to be in strict presence of the *Guru,* always being alert and having one's ears tuned to the simplest of instructions issuing from him.

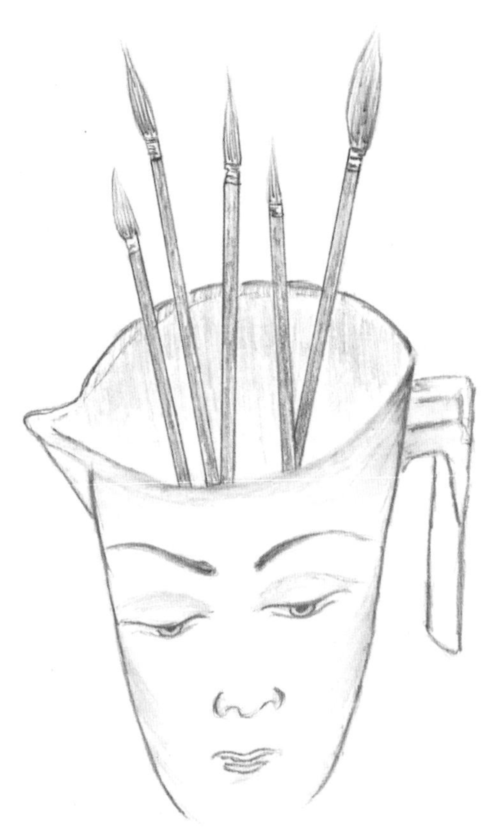

17 July 1997

Today, again, I saw a figure take something from my body and dash it on the ground. I saw various faces with different expressions. I saw my son's face. The faces end with a figure whose head is clean-shaven, upper body bare, piercing eyes, and with out-stretched arms beckoning me (like a mesmeric influence). I just keep watching – with the *'Om'* sound in me, my Brow *chakra* radiating a white fire between the figure and me. Towards the end of meditation, there is a form which starts radiating light from its Brow *chakra* on to mine. I can feel the pressure in my forehead. There is, again, a sound from the left foot like the hum of bees and the foot seems to twist.

18 July 1997

I see a number of mouths perked up in various shapes emitting rays and energy. I also see several pairs of eyes.

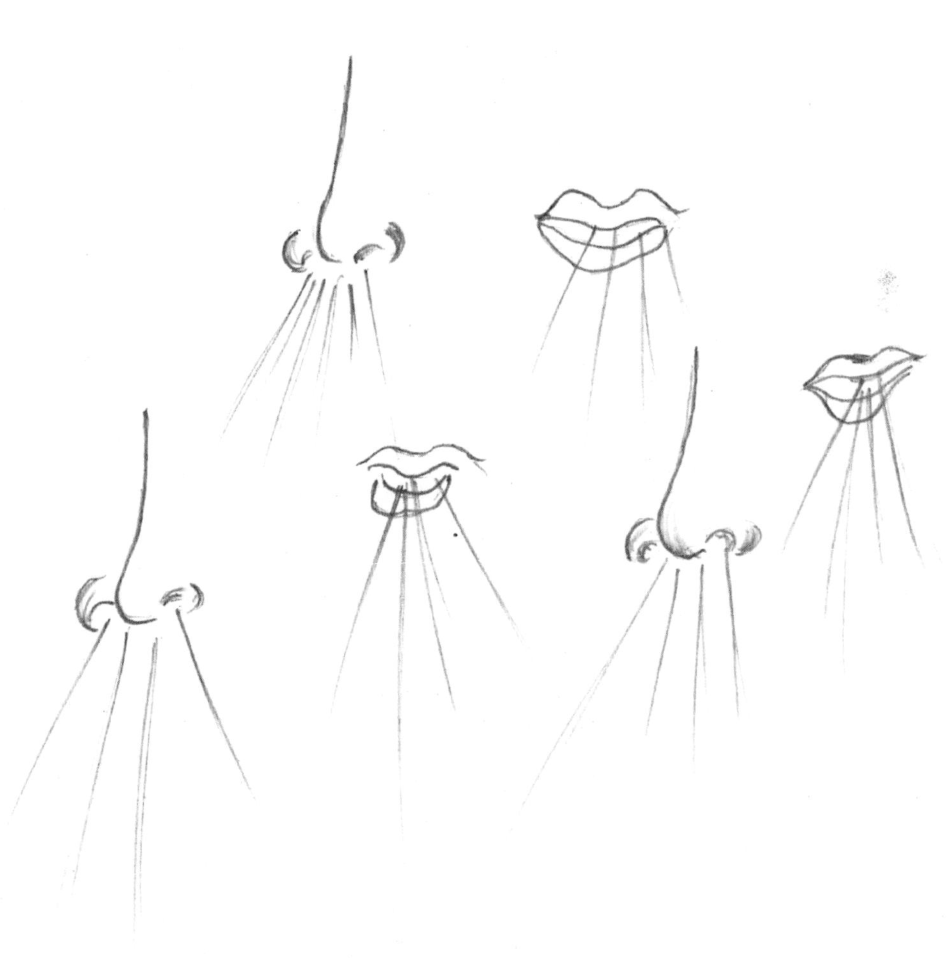

21 July 1997

I am moving at a speed where I become absolutely still. It is like turning a top or twirling a coin; the vision is not of movement but of me, absolutely stationary. Once that is achieved, it seems that I am the *Brahma chakra* (cosmic wheel of time), the size of a bullock cart wheel, gently rotating in space.

While meditating, my Self, from within, moved out and put a red *tilak* on my forehead.

22 July 1997

Group meditation at the Guru's residence: I am bottomless, clear water. Blue colour starts filtering in and I see my insides are as if white-washed.

23 July 1997

While meditating, I see myself going down on my knees and putting my forehead at the *Guru's* feet. The area around the *Guru's* feet is bathed in golden light.

"When this happens, when in the devotee's consciousness there is no place for his own thoughts or intellect an invisible flame emanates from the feet of the Master and it enters the brow-chakra, the occult space in the devotee's body. That flame then gives him all kinds of knowledge and the mind and the intellect of the devotee are under the power and protection of Shri Guru."

– Ashish, op. cit., p. 150.

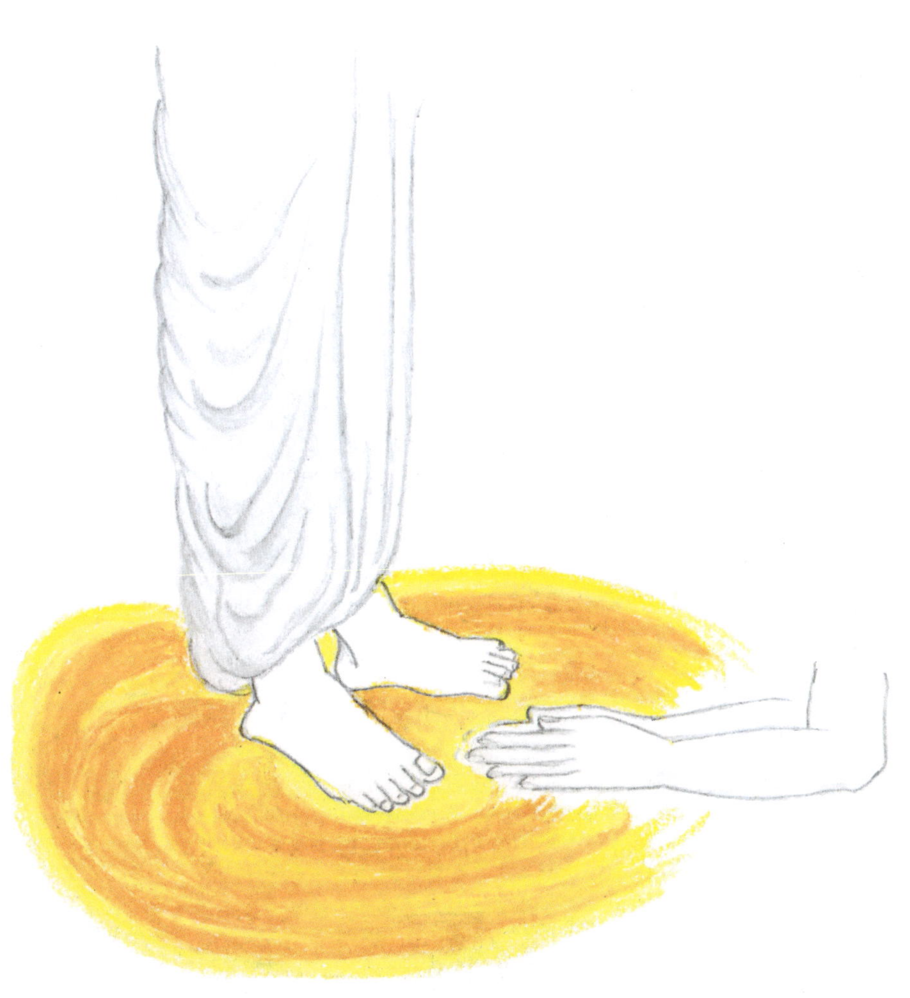

24 July 1997

During meditation, I am breathing in a particular manner; off and on the mouth blows up like a balloon and then deflates on its own; all very gently. I am not sure whether I am meditating or sleeping. Occasional thought surfaces.

25 July 1997

Birds come and plant themselves on my chest; among them are a pigeon and an owl. *Guruji* gives me a stone – tells me to keep it on my left body.

29 July 1997

While in meditation, I see myself standing and I have a scarf tied around my head like *Shirdi* Sai Baba. There are people coming from behind me and they walk through me. The cycle continues. I am Whole, I am the All, I am the Source. Creation is moving through me.

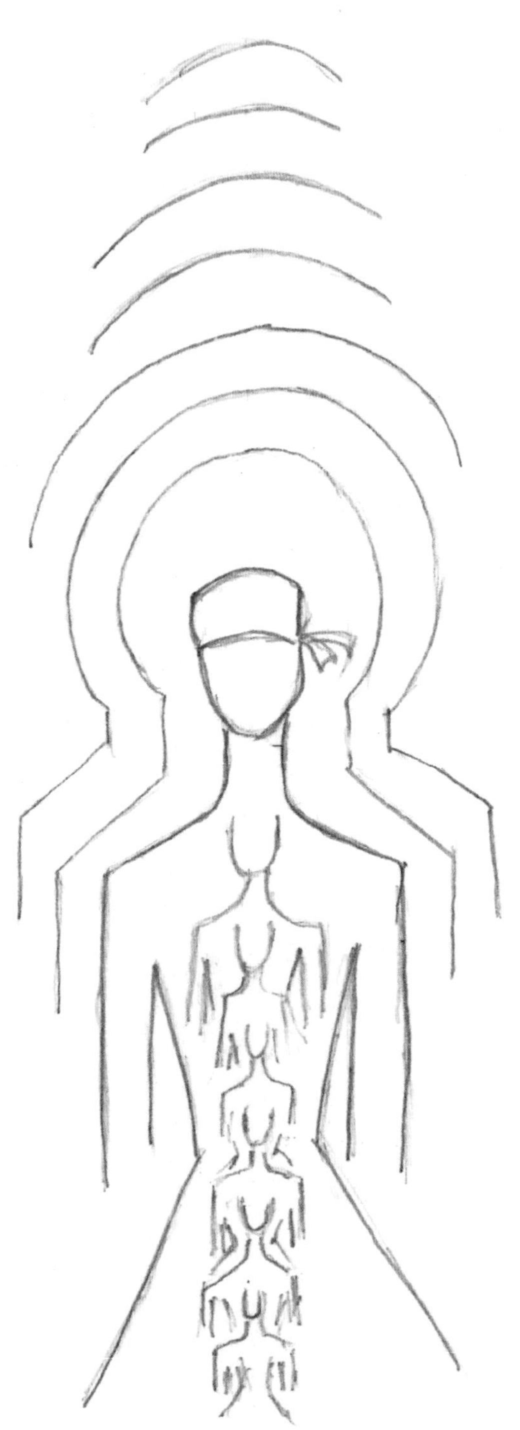

29 July 1997

Then, I see that I am moving around myself with my back towards me. I wonder why?

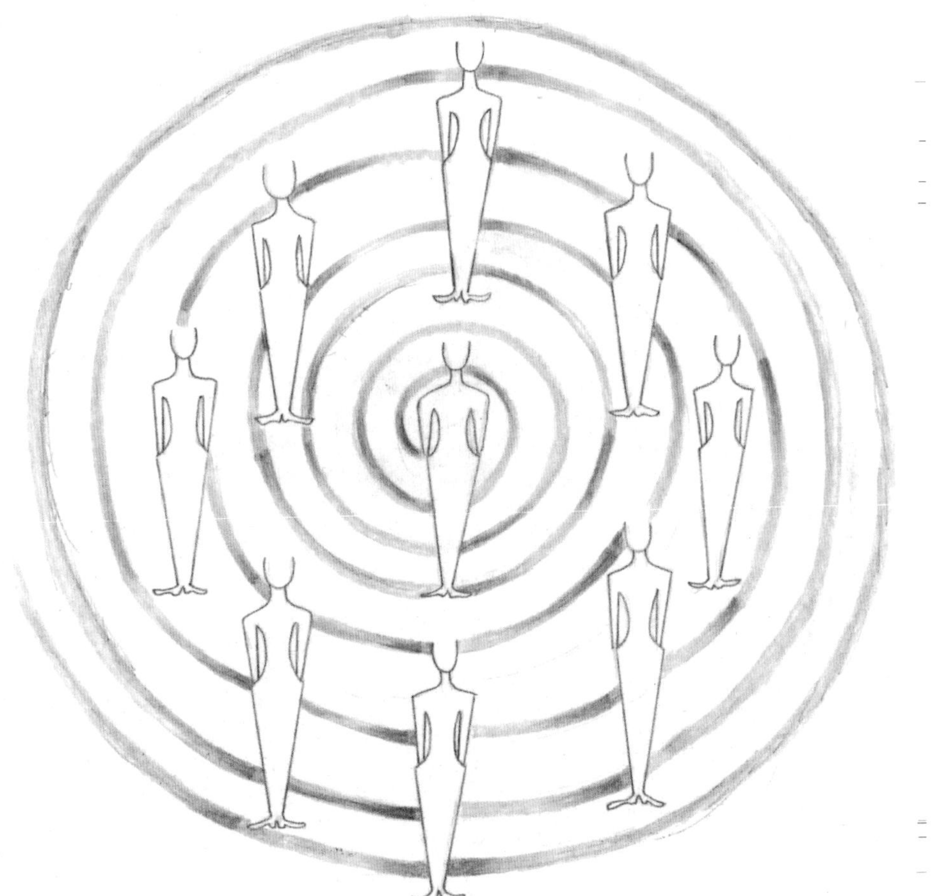

29 July 1997

I start to unwind as consciousness and then wind like a spring. Moving clockwise and anti-clockwise. The whole process is slow and gentle.

Group meditation at the Guru's residence: I was feeling very low. The sense is of being 'extinguished'.

> R. A.: The Spiral is back and she has been through a symbolic Creation-Dissolution process. So calmly had Santosh come to accept her meditative experiences that when something innately exhausting, like this experience, occurs she is nevertheless caught off guard when it tires her! To feel 'extinguished' in these circumstances is natural.

30 July 1997

The feeling of last evening continues.

4 am: During meditation, yellow flowers with *tulsi* are placed in my hands.

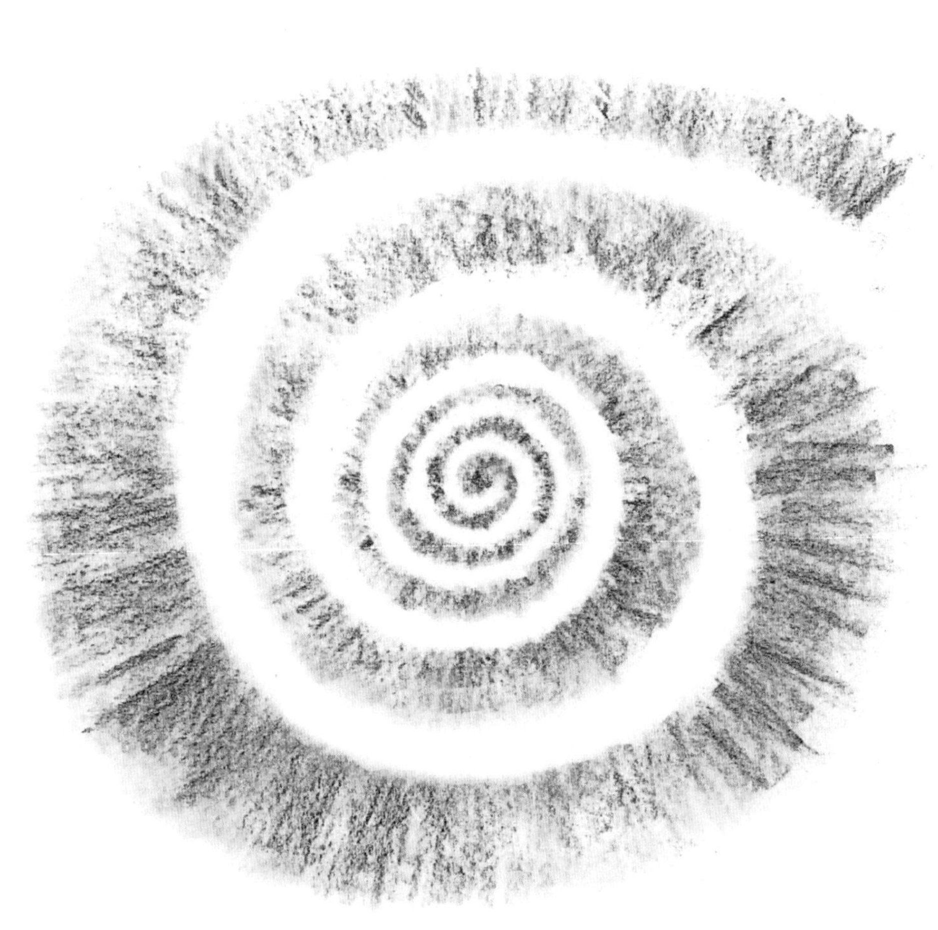

30 July 1997

I am climbing a ladder. As I climb the last rung, it breaks with a shattering sound. I break through a certain barrier and there is nothing else but blinding white light.

"Sushumna nadi is the direct line between mooladhara and ajna. It is the ladder connecting the earth and the heavens... That awakening is a historical event in the evolution of the spiritual personality of the individual."

– Saraswati, Swami Satyananda – 'Yoga Nidra'. Bihar School of Yoga, Munger, Bihar, India, 1976. Sixth Edition, 1998, p. 57.

R. A.: It is noteworthy, and Santosh has herself remarked on it, that the lights she has been in the habit of seeing have all faded and there have been only white light experiences for some time now. White light is, of course, an integrative quality encompassing within it all other colours in the spectrum. Her visions are becoming increasingly integrative; they are all being pulled together in a distinctly fresh direction from their free-wheeling range of the past. The reason why will be clear soon enough and the alert reader cannot miss it.

3 August 1997

Evening: There is a sensation of a cool, snow breeze blowing over the chest and the right leg. The meditation ends with the snowy coolness settling in the chest.

4 August 1997

My mouth opened wide and was getting wider and wider. The thought came that I wish I could see myself in the mirror. Not being able to do so, I did the next best thing and tried putting my fist in my mouth just to see how wide it was because it seemed as if an elephant could easily go in. Much to my chargin, I found that my fist was too big for my mouth. *Guruji* explained that it is the etheric body that expands.

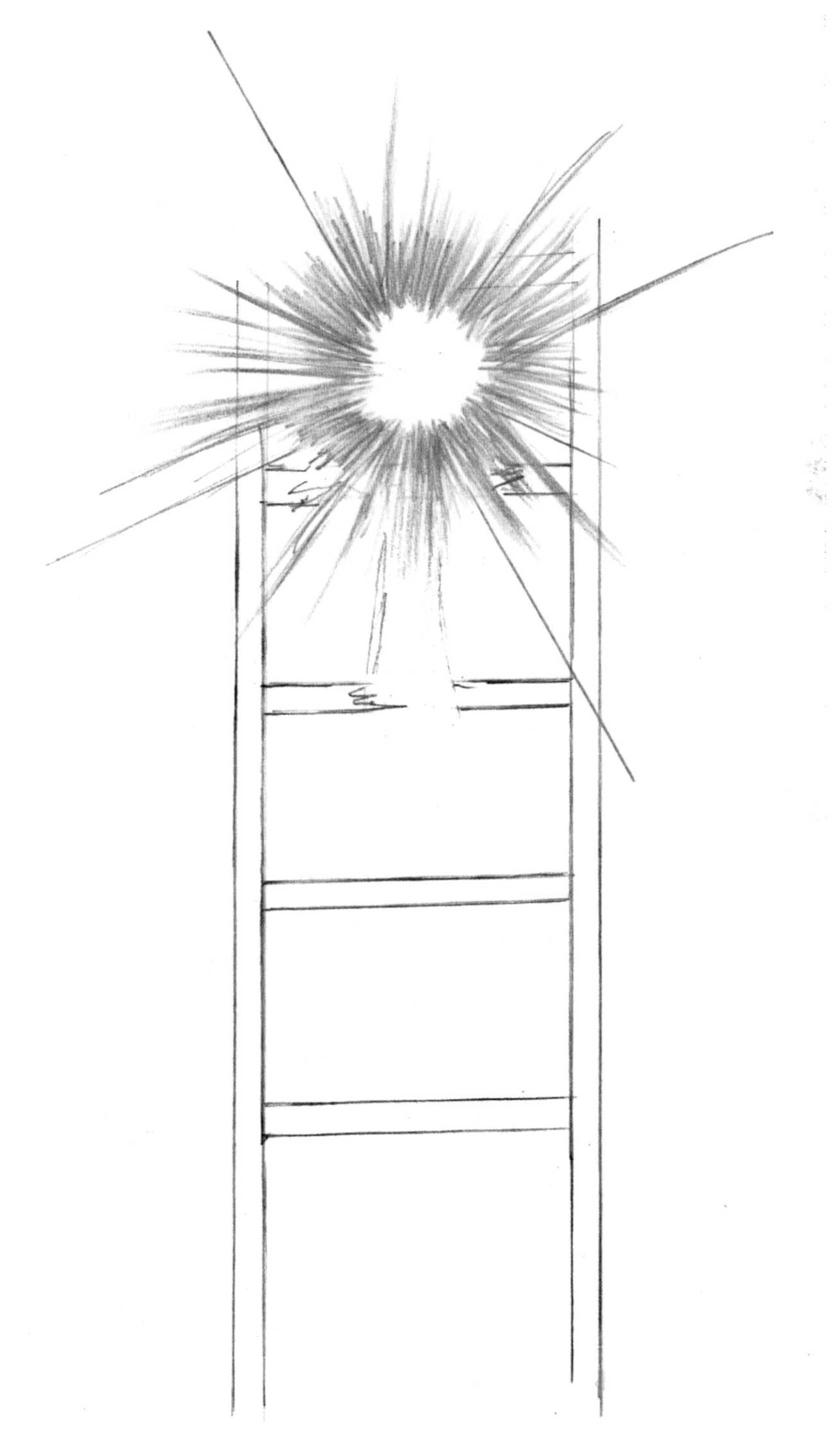

6 August 1997

I'm a drop, dropping in the ocean, partly merging.

I see a *rishi* in the water worshipping the sun.

R. A.: The *rishi* in the water is one of the most common archetypes of the Indian religious experience, it is also a religious practice that continues as a normal routine to this day. The *rishi* within the waters (of existence) symbolises the awakened consciousness literally seeing the light of truth.

6 August 1997

While meditating, I see a jumble of piled up thread unravelling very fast and moving into the void. At some stage, it disconnected and moved on, leaving the balance thread behind. To me, this represented the *Sutratma,* the Silver cord or the life thread. I realised that my life span was over as of this date and the balance life was a matter of Grace – probably to complete the work that was allotted to me to document and illustrate the working of *Kundalini.* On relating the above experience to my *Guru,* his interpretation was that it signified an end of the worldly life and a beginning of the Spiritual life.

"There is a silver cord which joins the physical body of a man with his subtle body. When you go out of your physical body, a silver thread comes out of your navel which joins the subtle body and the physical body, though you are travelling far away in that subtle body. Even if you go to the end of the universe this silver cord is intact and is not snapped... Death comes when this silver cord is snapped..."

– Ashish, op. cit., p. 256.

"...Those who are able to see in those lofty regions say that this form-aspect of the true man is like a delicate film of subtlest matter, just visible, marking where the individual begins his separate life; that delicate, colourless film of subtle matter is the body that lasts through the whole of human evolution, the thread on which all the lives are strung, the reincarnating Sutratma, the 'thread-self'."

– Besant, Annie – 'Man and his Bodies'.
The Theosophical Publishing House, Adyar, India, 1896. Second Edition, 2000, p. 107.

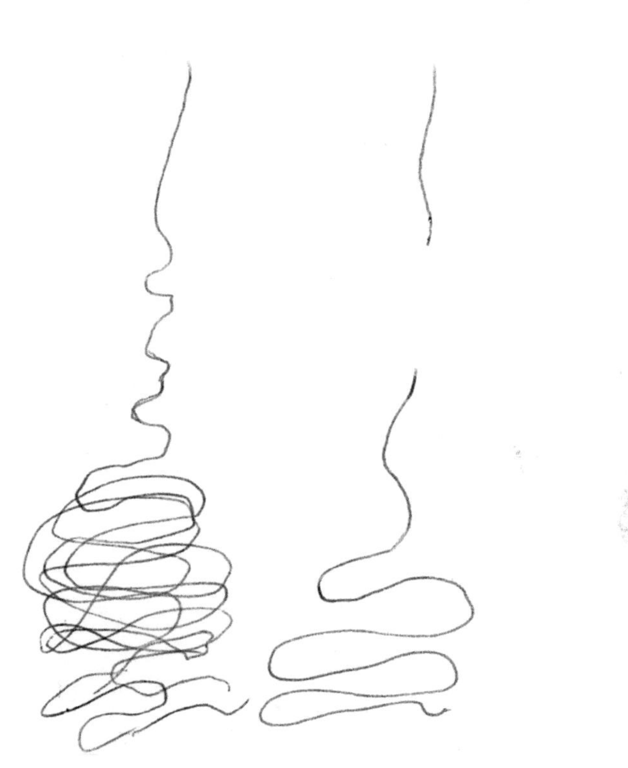

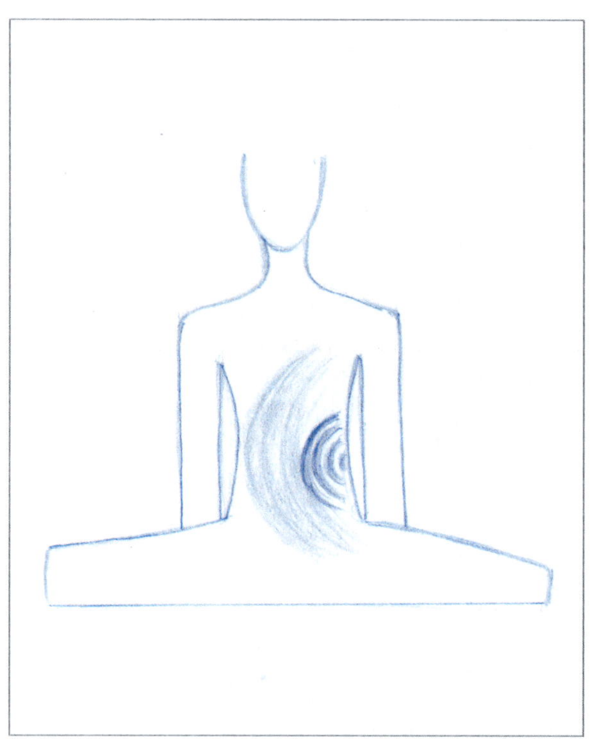

ENERGY BLOCKS & UN-EASE

My visual journey in self-discovery has lent a very clear understanding of the human condition as a whole. Our very physical form, and its appearance, is the result of our thoughts. Once we become conscious of this and understand the game, we realise that all that we have to do is imagine how we want to be and that is exactly how we shall be; we shall be self-created. As it is, we are following the Creation rules, but are doing it unconsciously. There is no system to our thought flow; there is a constant inflow of random thoughts, most of which have no meaning in our life, and we collect them and store them as junk data, thus causing congestion and traffic jams; jamming the flow of energy and thus compelling it to find nooks and crevices through which it can manoeuvre its way so that we can go about our lives in a reasonable state of well being. The best way to control the inflow of random thoughts would be to set the conscious mind as a censor to reactive thoughts, thus giving us an opportunity to act appropriately.

Un-ease before disease? How does it set in and manifest itself?

When does un-ease and disease set in? It is at times when we are not comfortable in any particular situation; when we are upset or our emotions have been disturbed through any negative feelings of hate, rejection, dejection, greed, revenge, resentment etc. If these negative emotions are not resolved and are harbored within our body-mind intellect, then, in time, this starts to slowly and steadily solidify and we set the process of un-ease, which would ultimately manifest as a disease in the physical body.

At first, it will start clogging and thus obstructing the free flow of *Prana*/energy in the subtle body meridians. This would be experienced as fluctuation of moods and imbalance in the trinity of physical, emotional, and mental dimensions. If an individual is following any self-development programme, then, through the process of meditation and self-analysis he will be able to resolve/dissolve the negative emotion that has taken the form of clogged energy. In this way, through conscious living, we move towards spiritual growth and prevent the clogged emotion from further solidifying and attaching itself to any particular organ to which the emotion is related.

The message is, 'we are the Masters of our destiny and authors of our death'. If we can live a happy, balanced life in harmony with the universal laws, without getting entangled in the inflow of random thoughts, we will probably move through life smoothly without causing an upheaval in the working of the system as a whole. Be calm, be cool, be non-judgmental, be non-complaining and non-reactive. If you can follow these simple rules, then you are living in awareness. Remember the 'other' has nothing to do with us. We are each creating our own script and drama, choosing our own cast, and allotting the roles to each as befits our psyche and who we feel are suitable to help us move through our growth and *karmic* patterns. Therefore, more often than not, there is friction in the stimuli and response in human interaction. For each is operating from the pre-inscribed script in his/her psyche. So wake up and be in the 'NOW', and don't live from past scripted patterns of stored data, and break your conditioning because it is hampering your growth and keeps you entangled in role-playing of the *karmic* game. Get up and get wise to the web that has been so intricately woven around you and get wise to the **play of consciousness**.

Once the realisation dawns, it seems so simple; what remains to be seen is whether we will be tempted and lured back into the exciting game of duality.

Chapter Three

BIRTH OF CONSCIOUSNESS

Ajna chakra is a point where the three main *nadis, Ida, Pingala,* and *Sushumna* meet. When focused at this centre, transformation of individual consciousness takes place. It is here that the individual ego merges with the cosmic ego and awareness expands and an individual enters the astral and psychic dimension of consciousness.

I marvel at the way a step by step process has been carried out with utmost accuracy and precision. With the *Ajna chakra* completely active, the atoms of the body rearranged, the spleen functioning at the subtle and physical level at its optimum, and the grace of the *Guru,* consciousness moves to scale a new map for Itself, demarking and determining the dimensions of space in which It would manifest.

8 August 1997

I have entered a new phase – there is a change in the flow and movement of *Prana.* The energy projects out from the *Ajna chakra* as a beam of light and moves in a very definite manner and in straight lines. The beam moves like a search-light starting the survey from over the head and moving in a downward arc.

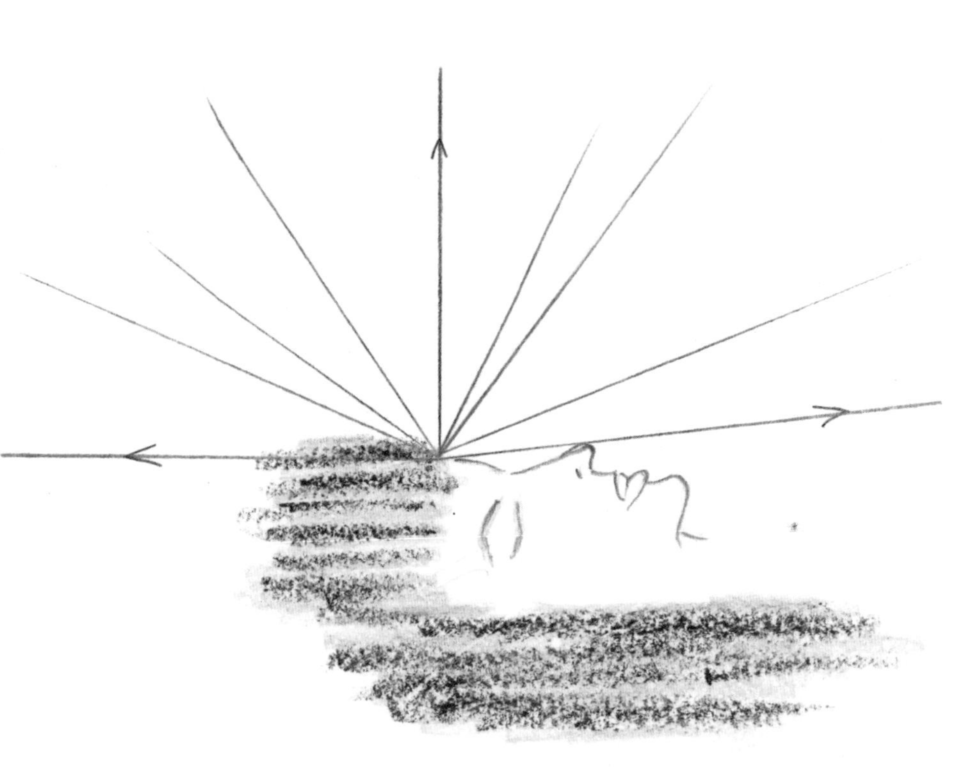

9 August 1997

From my right the beam now comes from outer space, moves across my forehead to the left, and then turns at an angle, goes straight up crossing through the *Ajna chakra,* through the head, and scans the area beyond.

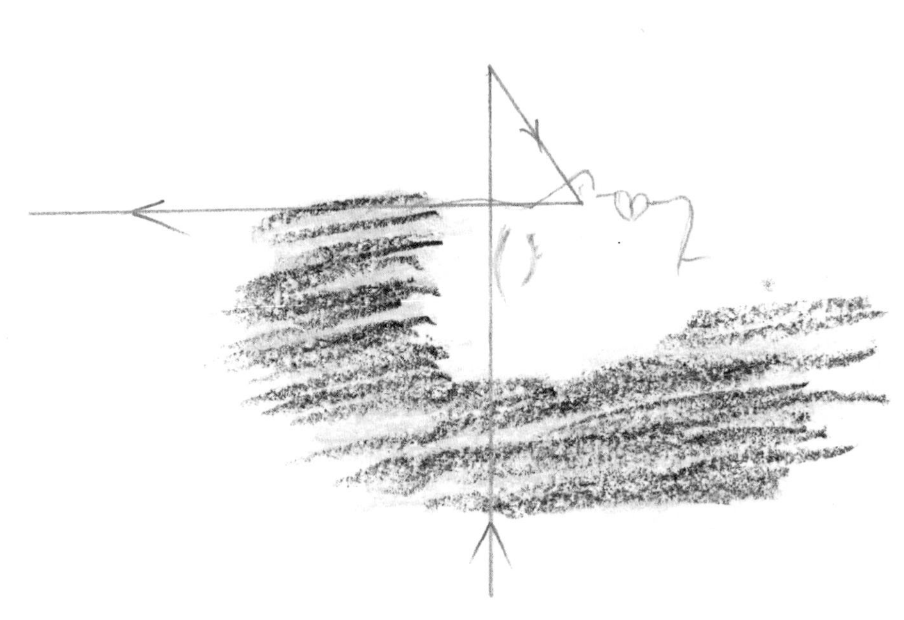

11 August 1997

The *Ajna chakra* gets fully operative as a beam in quick succession goes straight through the centre of the forehead to the back and through the head, filling it with a flash of light. This cobra head probably manifests when the *Kundalini* energy moves up and out in quick succession.

This exercise had to be carried out over two or three days otherwise the massive dosage of light would most likely have caused some short-circuits and damaged the delicate tissues in the brain.

> R. A.: The resemblance this has to the feathered headdress of the American Indians of the plains is quite strange.
>
> Whether it would be accurate to interpret the headgear as symbolic representations of expanded consciousness is not clear at the moment. However, it is to be noted that any old feather could not do in the making of these bonnets. They were constructed with the feathers of sacred birds only, totem animals perhaps, or spirit guides. A ritual and sacred context to the bonnet is therefore beyond dispute and it is not implausible to argue that they represent a different and superior stage of consciousness.

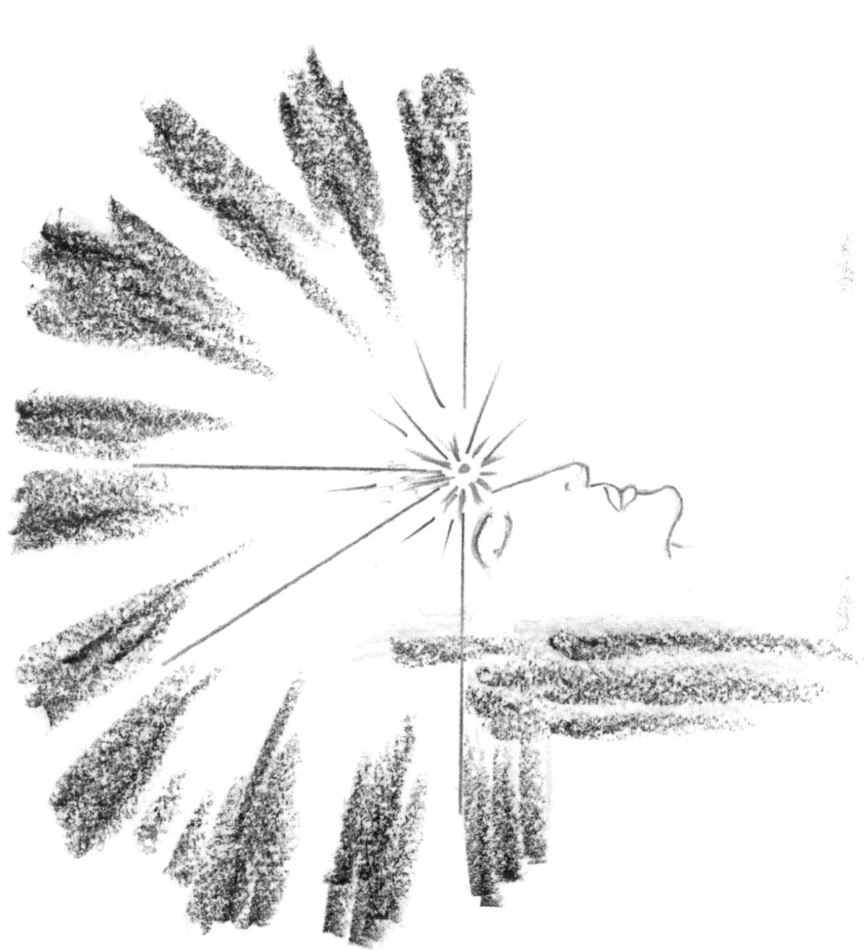

16 August 1997

Rays of pale blue light start at the feet, stretch over the body, and connect at fixed points beyond the head. I see my face in the front of the forehead, as in a small round mirror.

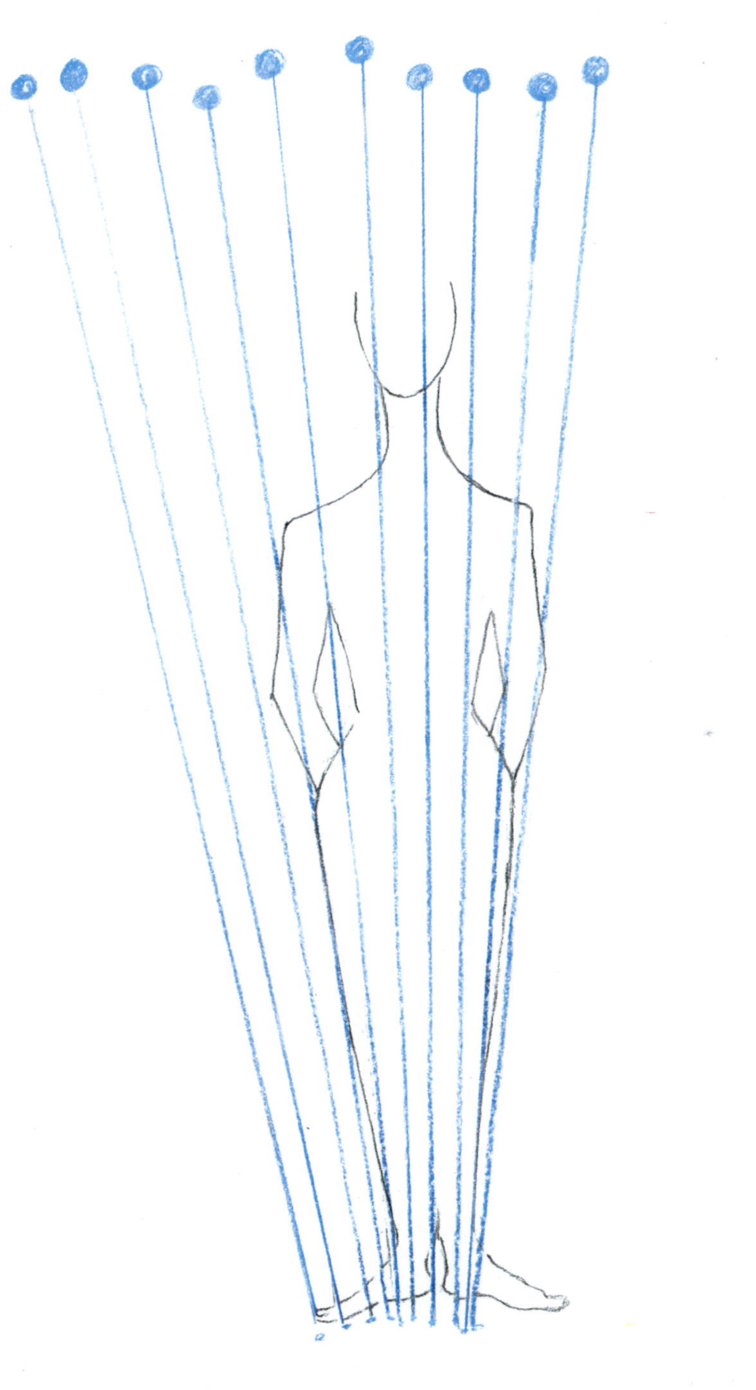

18 August 1997

From the right side of the chest, thick, etheric matter starts moving out till it starts merging with the cosmos. This is probably the clearance of residue of dense matter. I see my face in front of the forehead. Unseen hands bring a *bindi* in the shape of a half-black sun and place it on my forehead between the eyebrows.

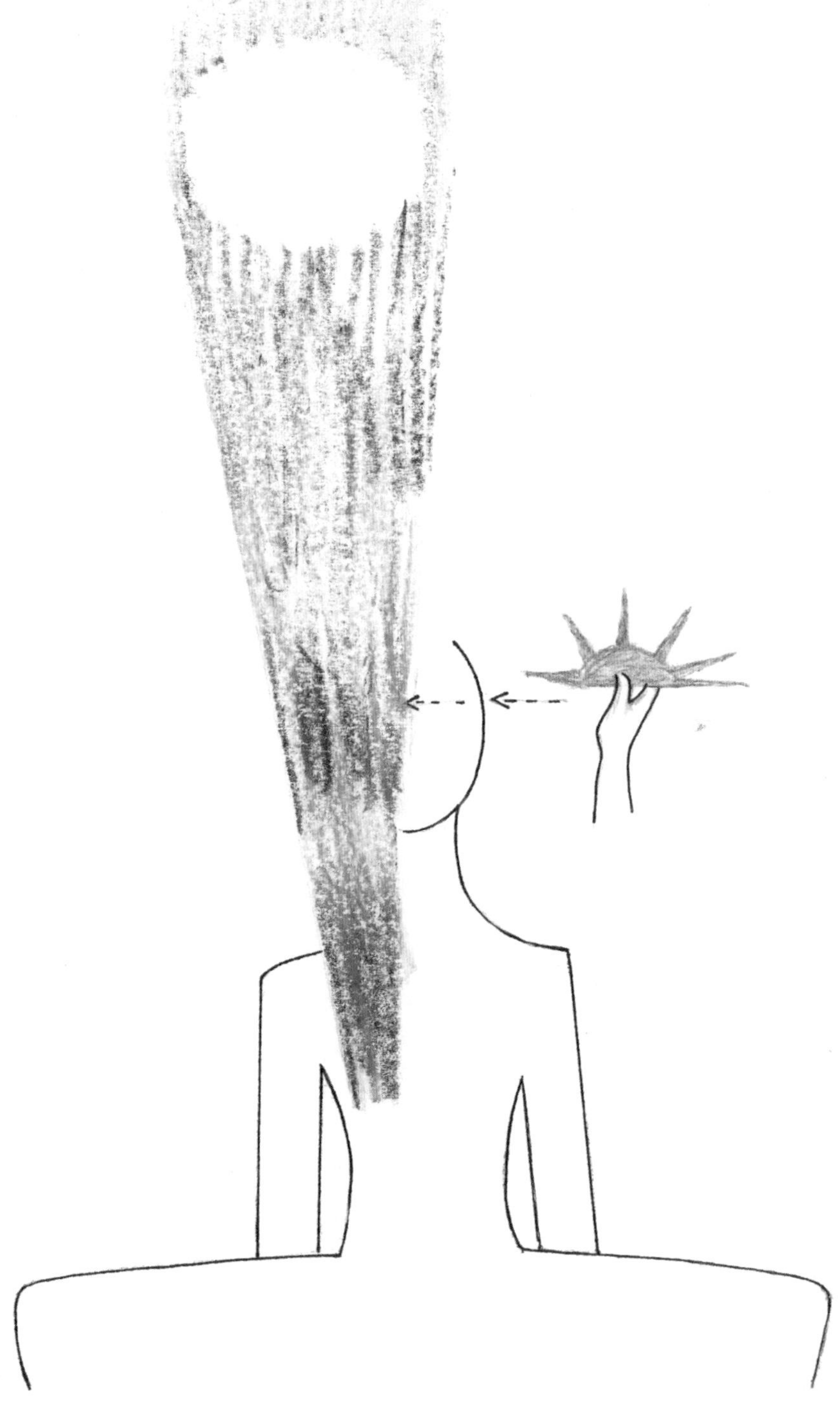

19 August 1997

A maroon-coloured flower blooms at the right side of the chest. Then the *Ajna chakra* in a funnel-like shape stretches and, extending, enters the flower. It elongates, stretches further, and re-enters itself, giving me the feeling of going deep within myself.

> R. A.: All flowers are, by their very nature, symbols of wombs and rebirth. It is interesting that this flower should manifest itself after the thick mass of etheric matter was purged from the body on the right side, on the 18th. What is even more interesting is that on the 21st she distinctly asks the question, "Am I in a womb?" The three states are closely interconnected and represent ongoing stages of a process of rejuvenation and rebirth.

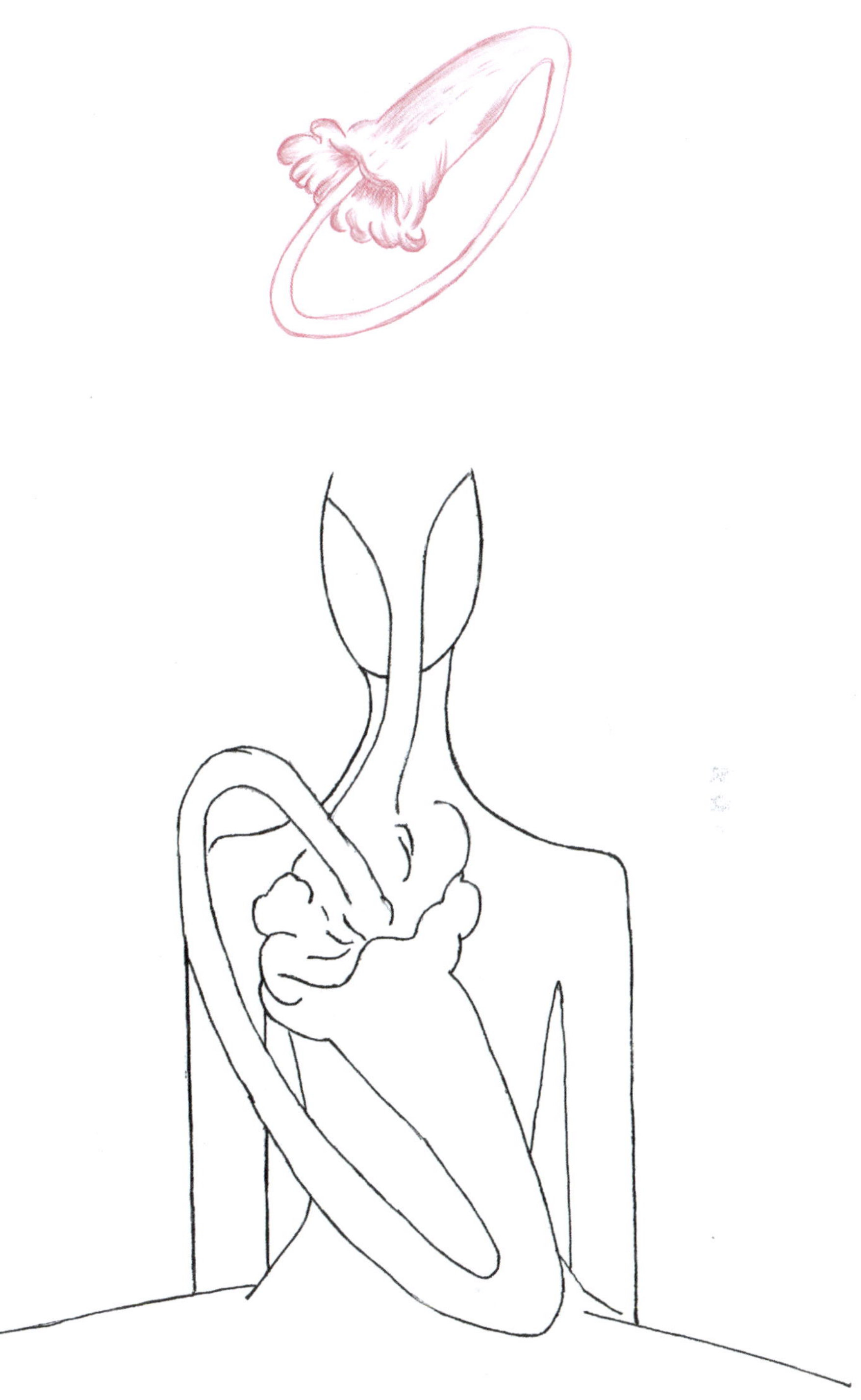

21 August 1997

I am in a state where I don't know whether I am in meditation or asleep. I see water trickling from the void till I am floating in it. It is a thick, transparent liquid with small bubbles in it, which reminds me of glycerine. "Am I in a womb?"

23 August 1997

My whole body is bathed in golden light. I see two jugs pouring golden liquid into my head.

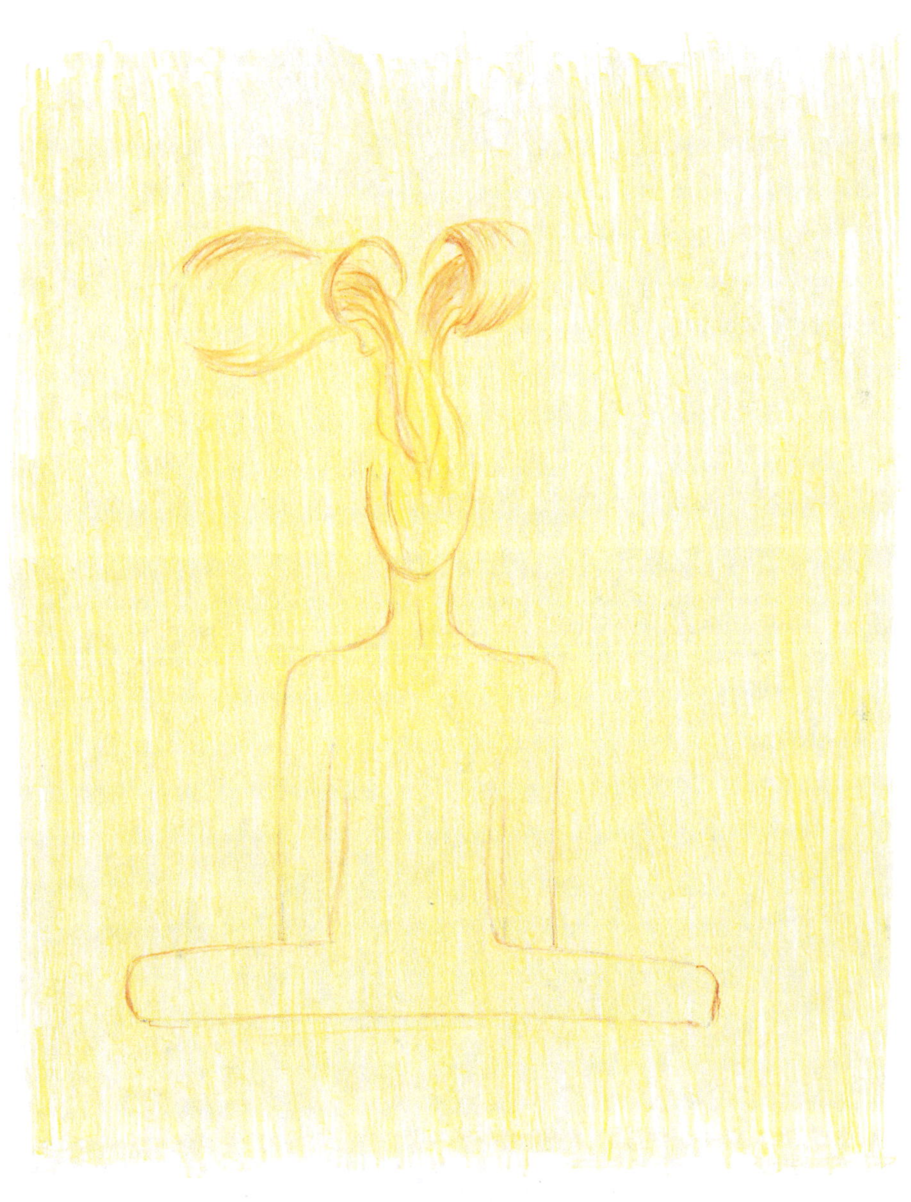

23 August 1997

The *Ajna chakra* elongates and moves within the body. It moves in different directions, surveying its deepest regions. The extended and elongated *chakra* looked like an elephant's trunk and it gave me an insight as to how *Ganpati* got his form. This meditation further activated my *Ajna chakra,* the source of all knowledge.

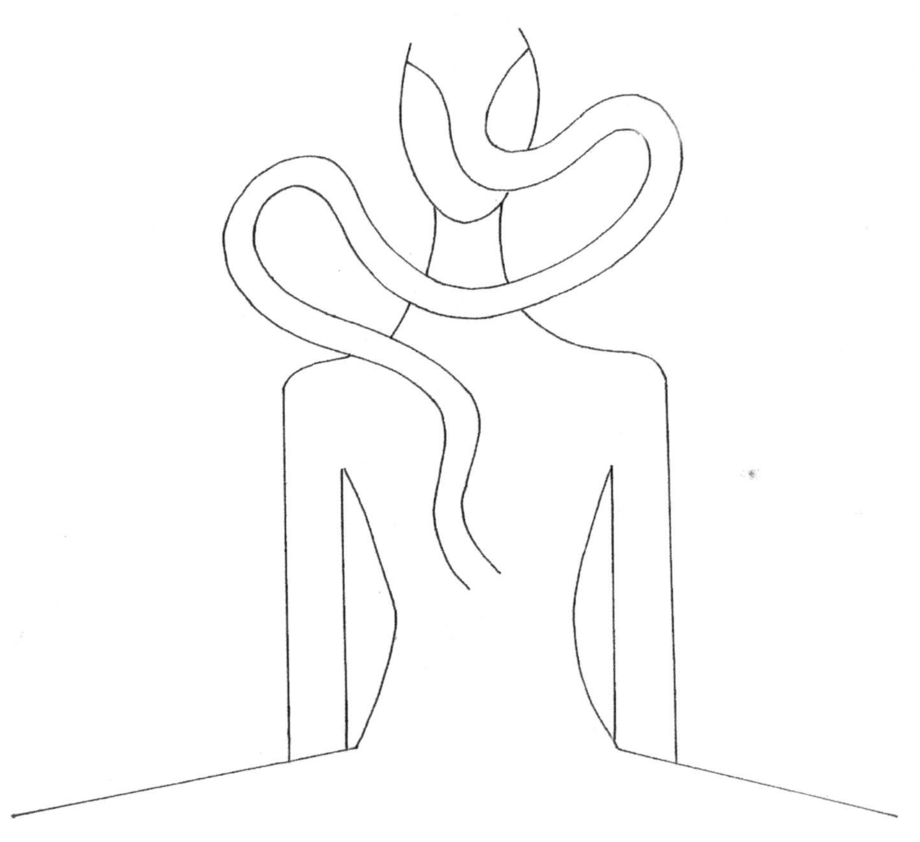

25 August 1997

The *Manipur chakra* became fully open and active, with the result I felt that my stomach was expanding to an unusual dimension. The *chakra* extended and elongated and, becoming a powerful beam of white light, started moving inwards and upwards till it came out of the forehead in bright, white, blinding light.

"Like the elephant's trunk, the discriminative faculty of an evolved intellect should be perfect so that it can use its discrimination fully in the outer world for resolving gross problems, and at the same time, efficiently employ its discrimination in the subtle realms of the inner personality layers."

– Nityanand, Swami – 'Symbolism in Hinduism'. Central Chinmaya Mission Trust, Mumbai, India, 1983. Third Edition, 1993, p. 142.

"His intellect must have such depth and width in order to embrace in his vision the entire world-of-plurality. Not only must he, in his visualisation, embrace the whole cosmos, but he must have the subtle discriminative power (viveka) in him to distinguish the changing, perishable, matter-vestures from the Eternal, Immutable, All-Pervading Consciousness, the Spirit. This discrimination is possible only when the intellect of the student has consciously cultivated this power to a large degree of perfection."

– Nityanand, ibid., p. 142.

The above experience makes me strongly believe that the ancient Sages, seeing the workings of the *Ajna chakra* and its acute wisdom and discriminative faculties, gave the form to the *Ajna chakra* the way it presents itself in combination with the *Manipur chakra.* The big ears of *Ganpati* are the vibrations emanating from the *Ajna chakra.* Coincidentally, the vibrations, expansion and extension of both the *chakras* when put down in the form of illustration, gives us the form of *Ganpati.* For further knowledge to unfold and my own evolution at the spiritual and material level to happen, the discriminating faculty monitored by the *Ajna chakra* and the material brain monitored by the *Manipur chakra,* both had to function in unison.

There is no way I can express my gratitude except to surrender in all humility to the workings of Source.

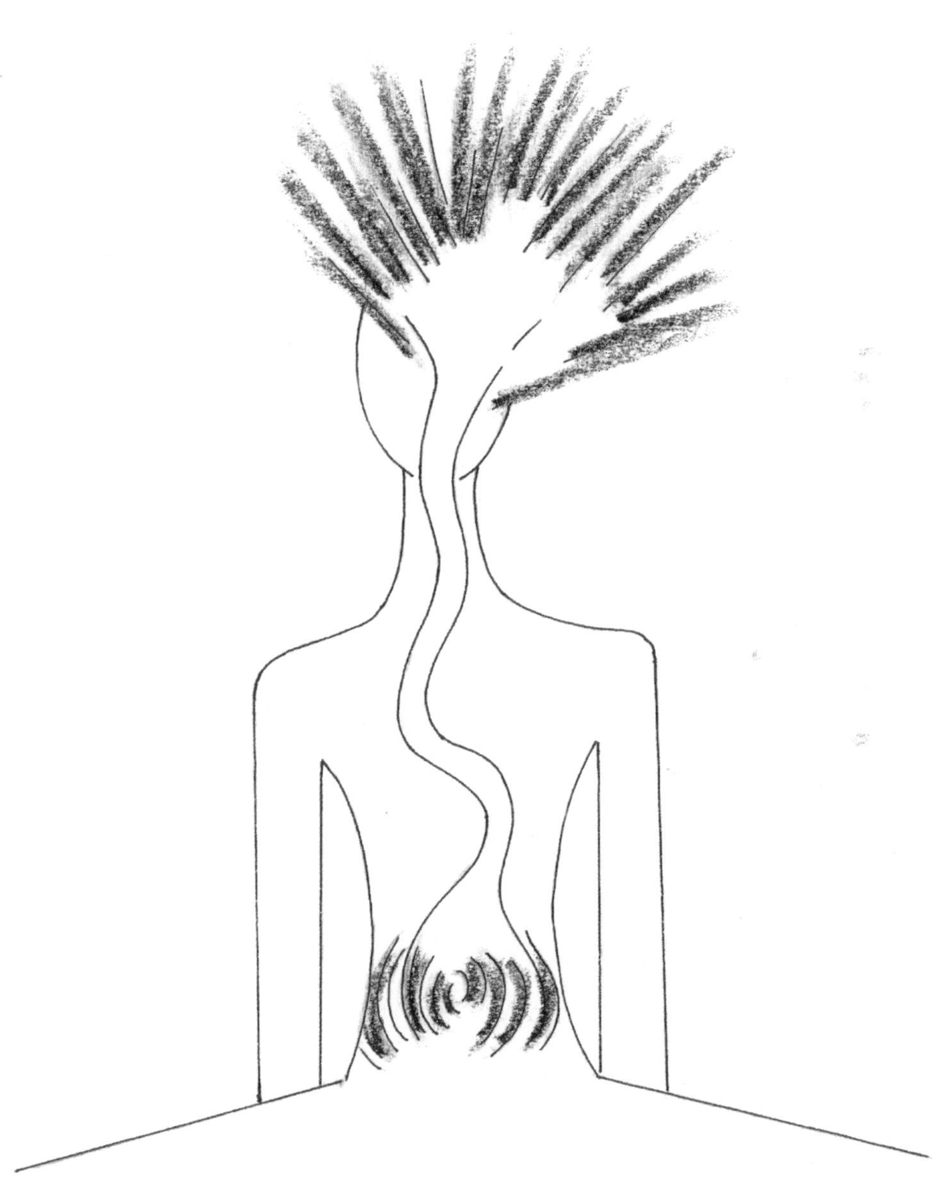

26 August 1997

The *Manipur chakra* goes deep within itself and above into space. The centre then starts spreading around itself into a sea of a thick, dark liquid. The centre is like a pole churning it. It brings to my mind the story of the *Amrut Manthan*. In the physical world the *Manipur chakra* is the centre experiencing life to its fullest. All emotions and ambitions are emanating and seeking fulfilment in this centre. Then, I move as light out of the *Ajna chakra* at a timeless speed and settle in the right of the chest.

R. A.: *Amrutha Manthan* – one of the core Indian myths where the gods churned the Cosmic Ocean so that the nectar of immortality, *Amrutha*, could surface from its depths. It is an instinctive cultural response to churning, so deeply imprinted on the Collective Consciousness is it.

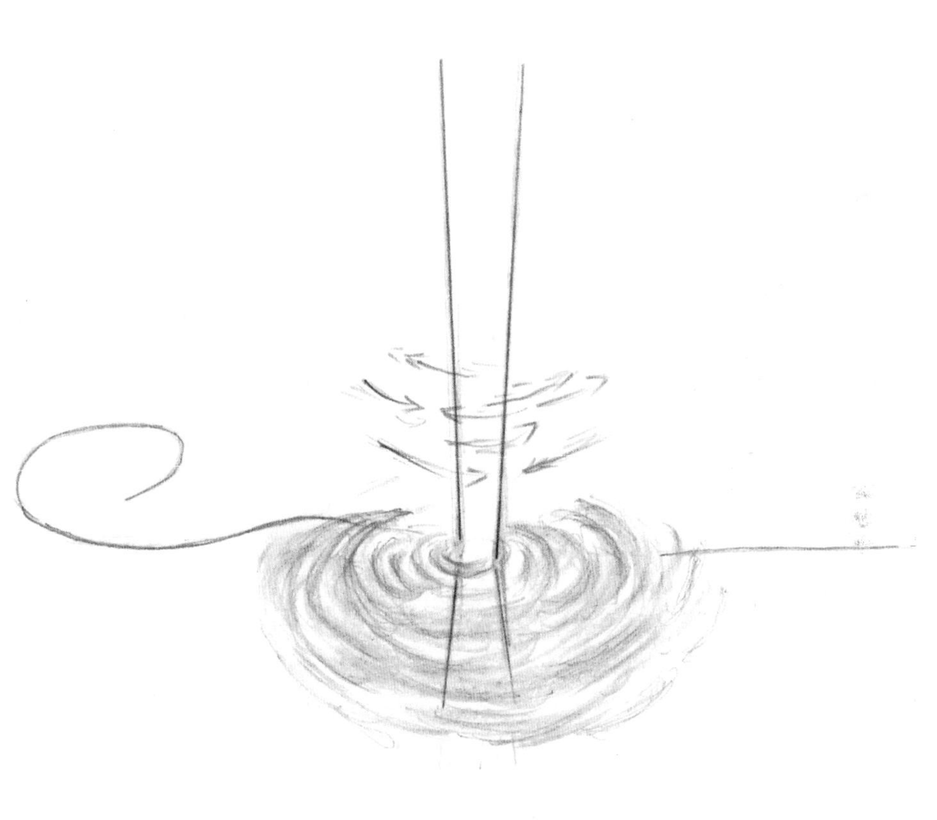

27 August 1997

After I had shown *Guruji* the visual of 18th August, he suggested that I paint a black circle, 8 to 10 cm, and practice gazing at it, starting with two minutes and then slowly extending the period. I found this exercise quite interesting. What I saw was that the black sun would start to change into a reddish glow. Next day, I saw what looked like a yellow flower in it. Subsequently, it divided into two suns, one black and one yellow; I would see both simultaneously till, finally, it settled back into a black sun.

Once that process was complete, I started to see a variety of human faces in the black circle, some pleasant and some not so pleasant. What was fascinating was that I would also see a face of a wolf and a horse. I figured, maybe these were the faces of my previous births.

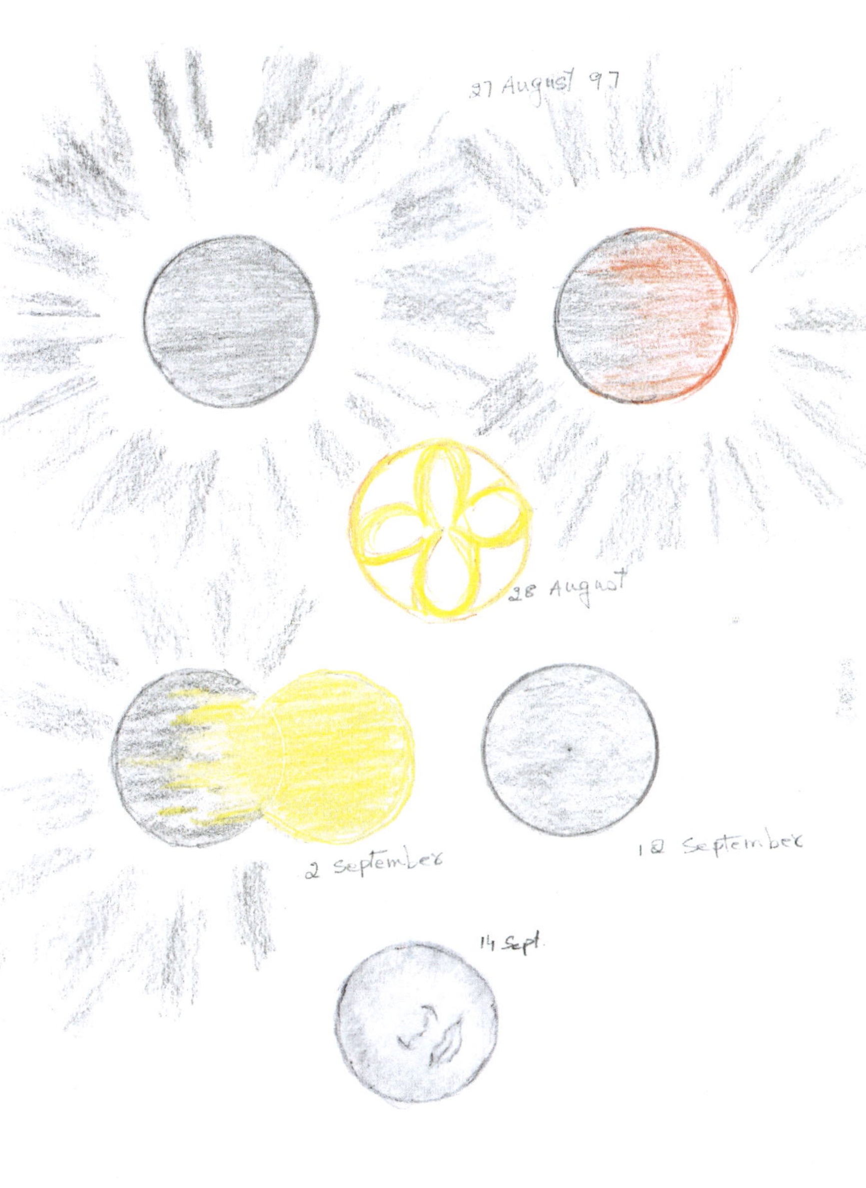
27 August 97
28 August
2 September
12 September
14 Sept.

15 September 1997

Today was special. A connection was made. I am the Milky Way. Now where I am, there is no rush, no urgency. I move as my nature is to keep moving. Smoothly supporting, carrying in my wake the universe, I am Energy. I am *Prana*. I am Consciousness.

17 September 1997

The sensation in my toes during meditation is intense, bordering on the painful.

19 September 1997

It is not an out-of-body experience – or moving out. It is more as if the body elongates from the toes upwards, with the feeling moving on to the torso, chest, and then the head. It is all very gentle and slow.

20 September 1997

3:30 am: I went to the balcony to look at the sky. I saw a most magnificent ring around the moon which, looking from the earth, was at least a kilometre in diameter.

I wonder:
Who am I? What am I?
I just am
I am movement
I am *Prana*
I am energy
I am constantly flowing

1 October 1997

I am at a well of thick, black oil at the chest region. A massive tube is pouring more oil into it. My ear starts extending; another massive tube is pouring more black oil – until I become a sea of oil. It is a dense sea, and movement is strained. I wonder what vibratory level this is?

11 October 1997

The crawling feeling is in the left shoulder blade. An electric needle rotating and throwing sparks gives a sort of an injection in the leg below the left knee. Light travels up the body giving a feeling of the left side separating from the right, bringing with it nausea and a lot of retching.

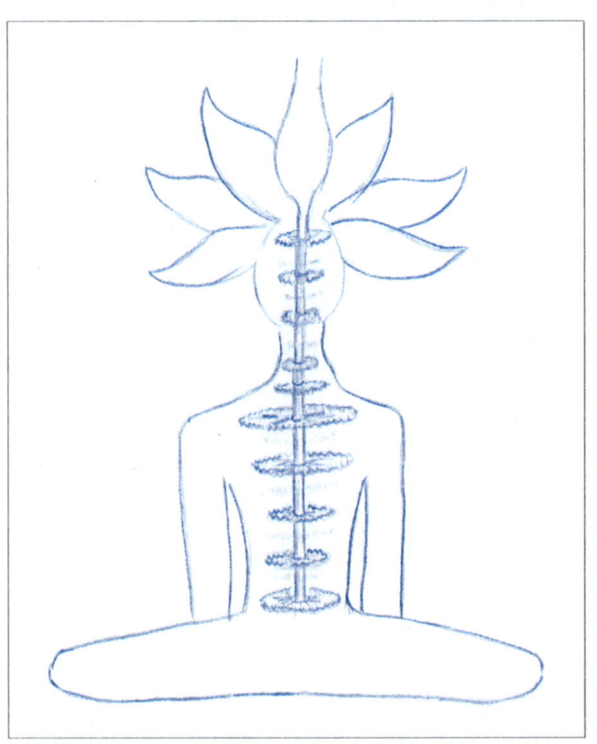

CHAKRAS

To consciously awaken *Kundalini,* the body-mind intellect is prepared through different forms of *yogic* techniques of *asanas, pranayama, Kriya yoga,* and meditation. When *Prana* is directed into the seat of the *Kundalini,* the energy wakes up and makes way through the *Sushumna nadi,* in the central nervous canal, to the brain. As *Kundalini* ascends, it passes step by step through each of the *chakras,* which are interconnected with normally dormant areas of the brain.

Step by step does not mean linear upward sequence from *Muladhar* to *Sahasrar* – the *chakra* that needs activation is activated. Although *Kundalini* is said to reside in the *Muladhar chakra,* we are all at different stages of evolution, and in some of us *Kundalini* may have already reached *Swadhisthan, Manipur,* or *Anahat chakra*. If this is so, whatever *sadhana* we do now might start an awakening in *Anahat* or some other *chakra.*

Once the multi-petalled lotus of the *Sahasrar,* the highest centre of the brain, opens up, a new consciousness dawns. Our present consciousness is not independent, as the mind depends on the information supplied by the senses. However, when the super-consciousness emerges, experience and knowledge become completely independent. The help of the sense organs such as the ears, eyes, nose etc. are not required. We see and sense what the physical eyes cannot see, hear the sounds which the ears cannot hear, get the fragrance which the nose cannot smell, and feel the warmth of the embrace that no body can match.

The Seven main *Chakras* and their corresponding Talents and Traits

Each of the seven main *chakras* has its counterpart in the physical body in the form of vital organs. The efficient functioning of these physical organs depends upon the functioning of the *chakras,* which are located in the subtle body. The more congested a *chakra,* the denser the related organ. Congestion of the *chakra* is related to the physical, mental, and emotional baggage an individual body-mind organism carries throughout its evolution. Therefore, the *chakras* not only control and energise the physical body but also control and affect the individual's emotional and mental body.

The *chakra* can change its size, shape, and movement according to the situation. The movement can change from rhythmic to chaotic. It can move like a flipped coin, up and down; like the pendulum of a clock, it can move clockwise or anti-clockwise. The rhythm changes according to the circumstance, situation, or mood. It's the rhythm and vibration of the *chakra* that indicates whether the event is related to a person, place, or thing.

"Awakening of the chakras is a very important event in human evolution. It should not be misunderstood for mysticism or occultism, because with the awakening of the chakras, our consciousness and our mind undergo changes. These changes have significant relevance and relationship with our day-to-day life... The higher qualities of love, compassion, charity, mercy and so on are the expressions of a mind which is influenced by awakened chakras."

– Saraswati, Swami Satyananda – 'Kundalini Tantra'. Bihar School of Yoga, Munger, Bihar, India, 1984. Reprinted, 2000, pp. 123-125.

It is contemplated that physical energy can be transformed into subtle energy through the actions of the *chakras,* and that the physical energy can be converted into mental energy within the physical dimension. As the *chakras* are activated and awakened, man becomes aware of the higher realms of existence, and also gains the power to enter those realms.

With joy and gratitude I present this vast knowledge in as precise and complete a structure as possible. I hope it helps all aspirants to understand the functioning of the body-mind organism. The best bet is to approach all our tasks in life with a playful attitude, finding humour and lightness in all situations instead of gnashing our teeth. Humour can lift us over the biggest stumbling blocks. A state of constant cheerfulness and always expecting the best leads us to new adventures and fulfilment. What I sow, so shall I reap. That is the cosmic law.

Muladhar (Base chakra)

Four petalled, deep red in colour. *Kundalini* is coiled here as a golden serpent, 3½ turns around the black *Shivalinga* in the centre.

Location: Perinium (midway between the genitals and the anus)

Element: Earth. *Tanmatra* – Smell

Sense organ: Nose

Importance: This is the base for awakening of *Kundalini*. *Brahma granthi* functions in this region.

It implies attachment to physical pleasures, material objects, and excessive selfishness. It also implies the ensnaring power of *tamas* –negativity, lethargy, and ignorance. This *chakra* is associated with monetary security and survival issues. Issues like feeling 'unsafe' in any given circumstance, and forever living under the fear of being abandoned. The related organs are the excretory organs like the rectum, urinary system, lower vertebrae, legs, and adrenal glands. The aspirant works towards bringing balance to his mental, emotional, and physical bodies, through self-analysis or self-development programmes. When balance is achieved, the knot of *Brahma* is released, the aspirant becomes centred, and images from the world of names and forms do not interrupt the meditation. The aspirant then moves towards increase in stability, a sense of connection with the earth, basic trust, self-confidence, sense of security, and then he moves in harmony with the laws of nature.

Mantra: *Lang*

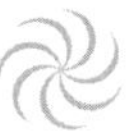

Swadhisthan (Sacral chakra)

Six petalled, orange in colour, with a crescent moon and blue waters inside.

Location: Genital region

Element: Water. *Tanmatra* – Taste

Sense organ: Tongue

Importance: In this *chakra* trickery, desires, and fantasies of sexual nature can be a problem. Instead of standing alone, an individual moves towards forming relationships and reaches out towards family and friends for physical contact. Restlessness and confusion are characteristics of this *chakra*. It is the store house of mental impressions. This *chakra* person pretends to be a prince or a hero.

Eating, sleeping, and sex must be regulated. The organs affected are the sexual organs and reproductive system.

Swadhisthan chakra encompasses the astral plane as well as the planes of entertainment, fantasy, jealousy, mercy, envy, and joy. The astral plane is between heaven and earth.

This is *Hiranyagarbha,* the universal womb, where everything exists in a potential state. Bringing balance between the mental, physical, and emotional bodies increases self-control, sensitivity, responsibility towards survival of the species, family, social norms, creativity, and solidarity with the surrounding world. One acquires the ability to use creative and sustaining energy to elevate himself to refined arts and pure relationships with others, having become free of lust, anger, greed, unsettledness, and jealousy.

Mantra: *Vang*

Manipur (Navel chakra)

Ten petalled, bright yellow in colour, with a blazing fire in the centre.

Location: At the navel (solar plexus)

Element: Fire. *Tanmatra* – Sight

Sense organ: Eye

Importance: It is the centre of dynamism, energy, will power, and achievement. This *chakra* radiates and distributes *Pranic* energy throughout the entire human framework, regulating and energising the organs, systems, and processes of life. When deficient, it is more like glowing embers of a dying fire rather than a powerful, intense blaze. In this state, the individual feels deficient in energy and lack of vitality.

A person dominated by this *chakra* strives for personal power and recognition even to the detriment of family and friends. Balance to this *chakra* is brought through selfless service or service without the desire for reward. The practice of charity will clarify one's path of action, or *karma*.

Meditation on this *chakra* awakens intensity and passion, essential for sound health and physical power. It gives powers of imagination, vision of the future, coming to terms with the past and desire for action. Concentration on the navel, the centre of gravity in the body, brings an end to indigestion and problems of the intestinal region. A long and healthy life is achieved. Fantasies are brought to practical form and one develops the power to command or organise. One develops control over speech and can express ideas more effectively.

Mantra: *Rang*

Anahat (Heart chakra)

Twelve petalled, green in colour, with a brightly glowing golden flame in the centre.

Location: At the centre of the chest

Element: Air. *Tanmatra* – Touch

Sense organ: Skin

Importance: It is associated with the bondage of emotional attachments and inner psychic visions. It is also connected with *rajas* – the tendency towards passion, ambition, and assertiveness.

It is the centre of feeling. *Vishnu granthi* operates here. With the development of love and compassion, love of life, joy, affection, unconditional selfless love towards fellow human beings, every creature, every element, and the entire creation, the knot of *Vishnu* is released and the aspirant becomes aware of his *karma* and his life's actions. His life becomes a source of inspiration for others as they find peace and calm in his presence. *Bhakti,* or faith, is the motivating force as one strives to achieve balance on all levels. This *chakra* encompasses good tendencies, and the planes of sanctity. The *Anahat nada* (cosmic sound) emanates from this centre in the form of *Aum*.

Mantra: *Yang*

Vishuddha (Throat chakra)

Sixteen petalled, deep blue in colour, with blue space inside.

Location: At the Epiglottis (adam's apple in the throat)

Element: Cosmos (*akasha*). *Tattva* – Sound

Sense organ: Ear

Importance: Evokes surrender, opens up the mystical dimension. In this *chakra,* purification and harmonising of all opposites takes place. It is the centre responsible for receiving thought vibrations from other people's minds. It evokes ethics, knowledge, expanded consciousness and complete harmony. One who enters the plane of *Vishuddha chakra* follows knowledge. All the elements are transmuted into their refined essence and only the subtle frequencies of the sense organs remain.

Mantra: *Hang*

Ajna (Brow chakra)

Two petalled, indigo in colour, sun and moon on the right and left petals respectively.

Location: At the eye brow centre (*Bhrumadhya*)

Tattva: *Maha Tattva,* in which all *Tattvas* (consists of *manas buddhi, ahamkara* and *chitta*) are present.

Importance: This is the centre where the solar and lunar energy synchronise; *Ida, Pingala* and *Sushumna* merge into one stream of consciousness essential for the flowering of awareness and concentration. Dissolution of duality takes place. *Ajna* is the bridge which links the *Guru* with the disciples. It represents the level at which it is possible for direct mind-to-mind communication between two people. Increases memory, regulation of all mental processes, rationale, intuition, inspiration, and memory. Here consciousness, superconsciousness, and the subconscious mind flow together. In the physical body it is the pineal gland. *Rudra granthi* functions in the region of *Ajna chakra.* It is associated with attachments to *siddhis,* psychic phenomena, and the concept of ourselves as individuals.

The solar and lunar nerve energies entwine up through all the *chakras* and meet at the *Ajna chakra.* This brings the sense of oneness and unity with the cosmic laws. The person realises he is an immortal spirit in a temporal body. The lunar liquid plane cools any excessive heat generated by the increased powers and purifies the conscience. *Bhakti yoga* maintains proper balance within the *yogi.*

Mantra: *Aum*

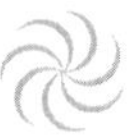

Sahasrar (Crown chakra)

Thousand petalled, violet in colour, with a bright golden *Jyotirlinga* in the centre.

Location: Crown of the head

Importance: Flowering of this *chakra* leads to a state of complete union with the Cosmic Consciousness or enlightenment. Here, one experiences a state of bliss and the Individual Consciousness connects with the Cosmic Consciousness. In the *Vedas* as well as the *Tantras,* this centre is called *Hirayanagarbha,* the womb of consciousness. It corresponds to the pituitary gland, the master gland situated within the brain.

In this *chakra, Samadhi* is the pure bliss of total inactivity. Up to the sixth *chakra,* the *yogi* may enter a trance in which activity or form still remains within the consciousness. In the *Sahasrar chakra* the *Prana* moves upwards and reaches the highest point. The mind establishes itself in the pure void. At this time all feelings, emotions and desires, which are the activities of the mind, are dissolved into their primary cause. The union is achieved. The *yogi* is *sat-chit-ananda,* truth-being-bliss. He is his own real self, and as long as he stays in his physical body he retains non-dual consciousness, enjoying the play of *lila* without being troubled by pleasure and pain, honours, and humiliations. Here the *yogi* becomes a *siddha,* but has transcended the desire to manifest his wishes.

Mantra: *Aum Satyam Aum*

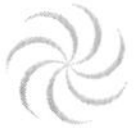

The books I used for reference are:

Kundalini Tantra by Swami Satyananda Saraswati, *Mudras* by Gertrud Hirschi, *Chakras* by Harish Johari, *Chakra Dhyana, a musical path to meditation* chanted by Krishnaraj Bhagavandasa, and *Kundalini Diary* by Santosh Sachdeva.

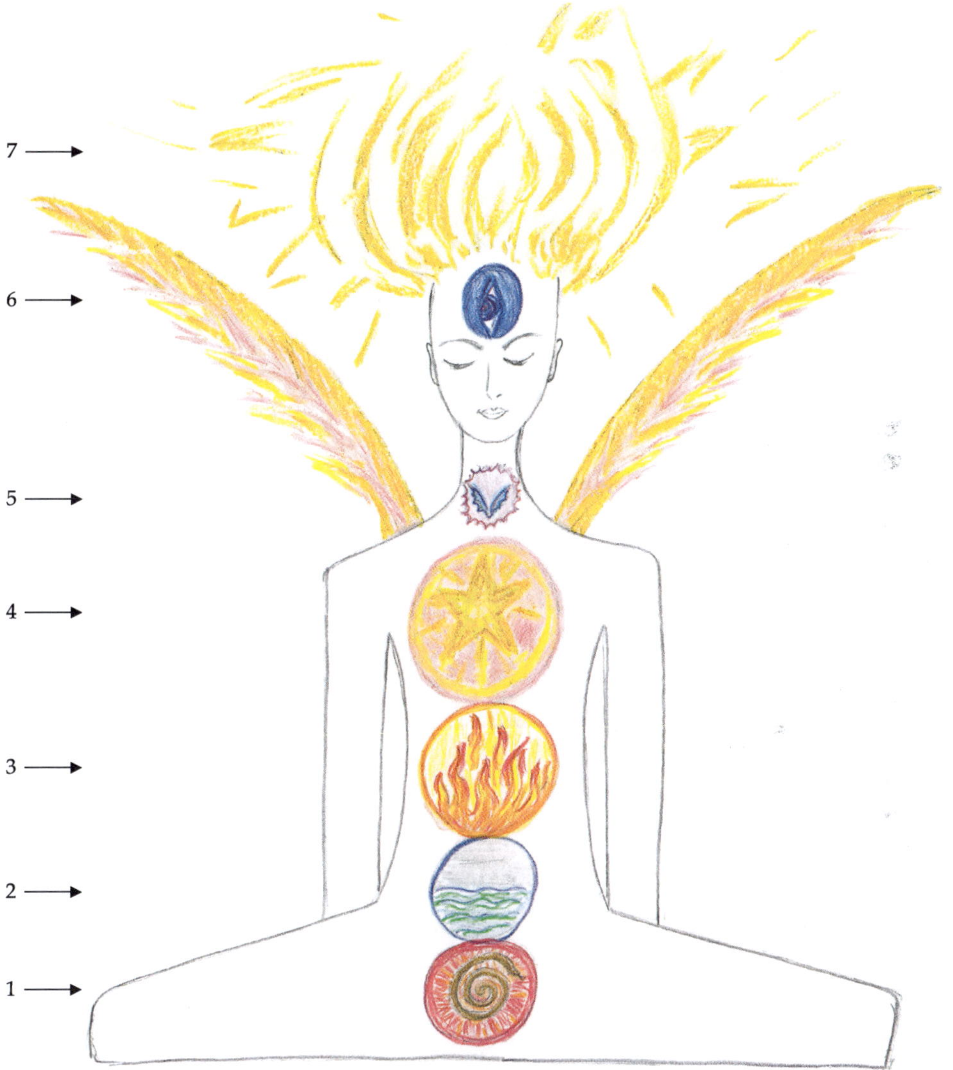

Chakras and the Body Temple*

1 – Muladhar (Base chakra)
2 – Swadhisthan (Sacral chakra)
3 – Manipur (Navel chakra)
4 – Anahat (Heart chakra)
5 – Vishuddha (Throat chakra)
6 – Ajna (Brow chakra)
7 – Sahasrar (Crown chakra)

**This chart showing the location of the seven main chakras in the etheric body is a stylised version created by the author, and the colours and symbols shown here do not necessarily correspond to the descriptions in the traditional literature on Kundalini.*

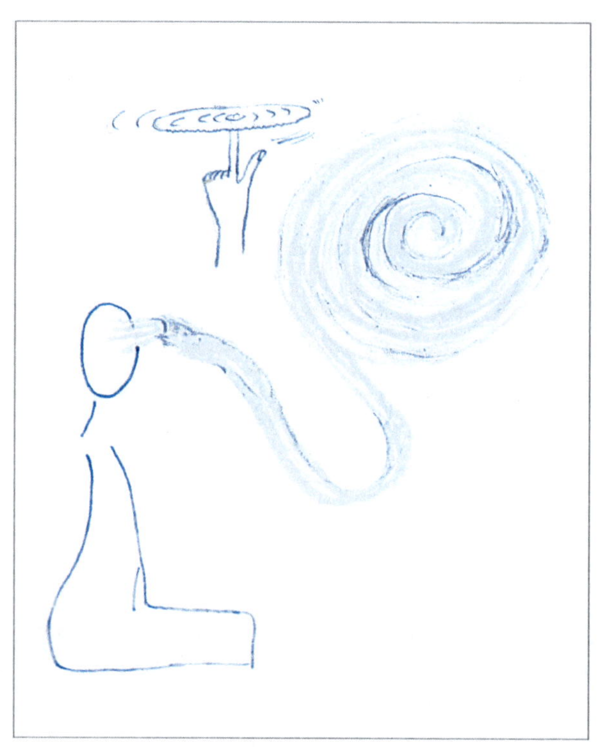

Chapter Four

KUNDALINI OPERATIONS

Swami Niranjananda Saraswati, in his book *Prana Pranayama Prana Vidya,* tells us that once *Ajna* is developed *Prana* can be experienced in the form of light, and its movement throughout the body can be visualised. *Ajna* is the point where the mind changes from gross to subtle, from outward to inward.

Manipur is a storehouse of *Prana* and is associated with heat, vitality, dynamism, generation, and preservation. As the sun radiates light and energy, so *Manipur* radiates and distributes *Prana* throughout the body, regulating and fuelling life's process.

With the *Ajna* and *Manipur chakra* working in unison, a new phase of learning and unfoldment of knowledge opens up (see visual p. 121, 25th August, 1997).

18 November 1997

Group Meditation shifts to my home.

Meditation had to shift from *Guruji's* place due to unavoidable circumstances. Since my flat is centrally located, I thought it appropriate to have the meditation at my place.

During meditation, I saw that *Guruji* was meditating with eyes open, and only the white of his eyes were showing. His head was turning in slow motion from right to left and left to right. It was awe-inspiring. I got the feeling that he was surveying the universe from another dimension.

28 November 1997

11 pm: I felt a presence moving over me. Then, it blew its breath onto my face. When I mentioned this to my Reiki Master, she said that the Reiki Masters send healing to their students.

❦

9 December 1997

During meditation with *Guruji* and the group, I felt an opening in the crown, someone blowing cool air into it, and cool air circling it. I also felt as if some light substance was dropping on the head.

1 January 1998

The *Ajna chakra* gets active and throws out beams of light, which extend over a vast distance.

Two beams of light intersect each other in the centre of the forehead. The upper two ends move inwards to form an elongated U, whereas the bottom ends move towards each other to form an inverted ∩; both continue to intersect each other making the centre look like an eye. This, surprisingly, looked like the *tilak* (ꟸ) on the forehead of the *Vaishnavites*, worshippers of *Lord Vishnu*.

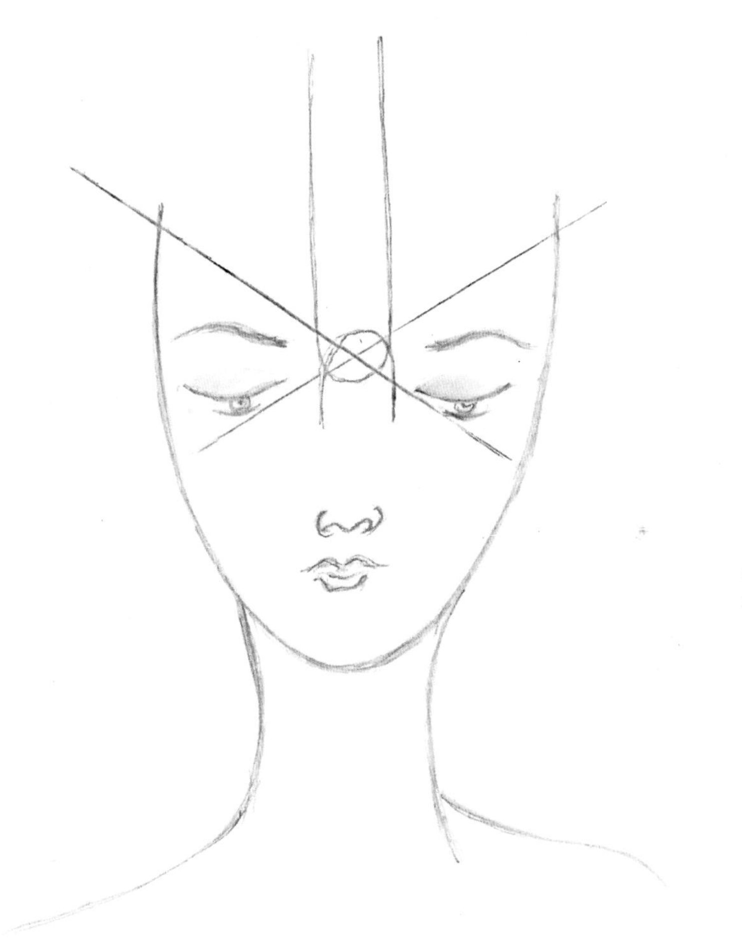

1 January 1998

The visualisation of the *tilak* raised my consciousness to a level where I found myself sitting on tiny waves, which looked like tips of petals (Fig. 1). After meditation, when I put the visual down on paper, I sat gazing at it and it threw up the impression of a lotus flower (Fig. 2). Is this the vibratory level where all manifestations take place?

Void, as I come to understand now, is the subtle form of water. No wonder then, that I see the vibratory levels as waves in their different patterns and denseness, and the lotus becomes the natural symbol for this subtle level.

Fig. 1

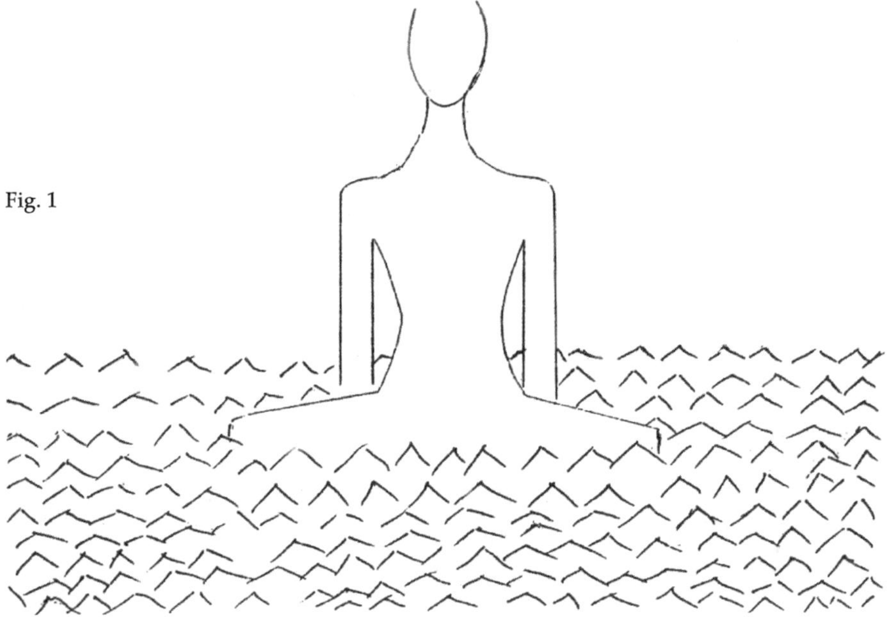

Fig. 2

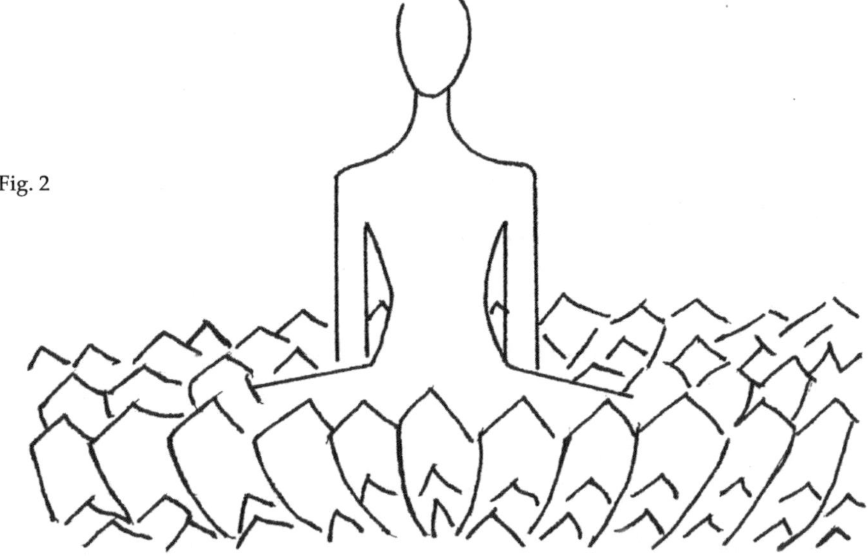

1 January 1998

Subsequently, my forehead gets fully illuminated and a band of white light runs across my forehead; the two ends move up leaving the centre as a bright flame, creating a shape of a *trishul* (trident), thus creating a symbol for the *Shaivites,* the followers of *Shiva.*

The realisation dawns, that in order to reach the subtlest level of *Shiva* consciousness my consciousness had first to attain the level of *Krishna* consciousness. If anyone had tried to explain to me the intracacies of different levels of consciousness, I would have found it impossible to comprehend. I find this the best way of getting any knowledge; knowledge without studying but through experience, awareness, and understanding.

In Hindu mythology, different aspects of the Abstract Principle have been given different forms based on the vibratory pattern of the particular level. The remover of obstacles has been given the form of *Lord Ganesha* with an elephant's trunk; wealth has been given the form of *Goddess Laxmi* seated on the lotus, and so on. These forms are given to the different aspects of the Abstract Principle in order to help an individual focus on that aspect of the Supreme Reality which he is in most need of and appeals to him the most. While focusing on the form of his choice, he is still focusing on the Abstract Supreme Reality – but without awareness. To him, the form becomes his God.

> R. A.: These visuals are interesting because they give clues to one of the most robust and enduring symbols of Indian culture – the holy personage visualised as being seated on a lotus. This is especially true of *Laxmi,* goddess of good fortune. One of her many names is *Padma,* the lotus. Santosh has written on the importance of these visions and their cultural context specificity well, but there is something equally important here. It is as though on one single day, 1st January, 1998, she was given an introduction to the thinking behind the symbolism of the three major strands of Hindu interaction with the divine – *Shiva, Vishnu,* and the most benign form of the Great Goddess, *Laxmi.*

I read somewhere: "Awakening is a universal process... only symbolism changes in relation to the impressions on the subconscious depending which culture one comes from."

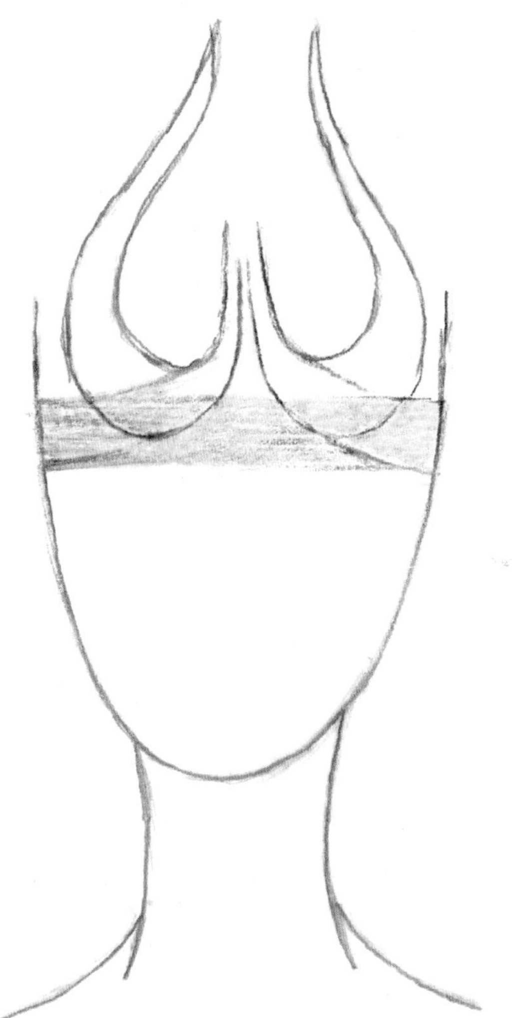

11 February 1998

Morning meditation: I see a flash of light, and what look like the *Devanagri bij mantra Hrim Shrim,* come towards me.

13 February 1998

I see a rainbow among the stars.

14 February 1998

A dog snaps at my left toe as if to bite it off. This is interesting in hindsight, because I have now become aware that I must have a *karma* related to lameness and continue to experience weakness, especially in the right thigh in this present life. As described in Volume I, the ankle of my right foot was saved from amputation when I was an infant just five or six months old. I've also had past life glimpses of a dismembered leg belonging to my body as a dead soldier.

16 February 1998

There is an explosion of a different kind in the head. There is a sensation of the brain being scorched. This is the repetitious experience of the destruction of old *karmas* in meditation, almost as if the physical body is going through the actual experience of cremation. The sounds of explosion recall the image of the skull bursting in the cremation fires, in different cycles of birth and death, while I work my way through old *karmas* during meditation, in the quest of liberation.

17 February 1998

I say "Hello!" to *Shiva.*

On my early morning walk, I see a young beggar with a head of thick, curly hair coming towards me. He is light of foot, has a mischievous smile, and is thoroughly alive for that hour of the morning. The thought that comes to my mind is – *where are his crutches?* For, he is the same beggar whom I have sometimes seen in my dream and on the astral plane while in meditation.

The sight of him makes me feel good and joyful. As he comes before me, he gives me a rakish smile and salutes. I respond with the same enthusiasm. The feeling of comradeship and euphoria stays with me for days.

"Sometimes the Lord will come before you in the form of a beggar or sick man with dirty rags. He may appear before you in the form of a coolie or a man of low caste. You must have the keen sense to detect him."

– Sivananda, op. cit., p. 326.

24 February 1998

Group meditation: I see the *Guru's* head as a skull, with dark holes in place of the eyes.

26 February 1998

I seem to be only aware of the inhalation of air while breathing, but not the exhalation. The process of breathing seems to be restricted to the area between the navel and the heart.

"Breath-control: There are many varieties of breath control. Kundalini when awakened, gets these automatically done."

– Ashish, op. cit., p. 247.

27 February 1998

It seems as if there is no brain inside my skull; in its place I only see a pale, golden dome.

1 March 1998

I see a *tulsi* plant. *Guruji* gives me some kind of a fruit, which is handed to me in a leaf.

17 March 1998

The silver cord burns at one end, which gets totally charred. This is a vivid depiction of the destruction of old *karmas* and past attachments.

2 April 1998

I see needles being put into different parts of my head, and I realise that I seem to be undergoing acupuncture treatment in the course of the meditation. Awareness returns with the insertion of the needle above the neck and at the base of the back of the head, on the left side. I also see my right leg in a prone position, supported by callipers.

It seems that all sections of my brain have to be activated, or that my awareness at all levels is required to function at a high level of efficiency, in order to assimilate what is to come.

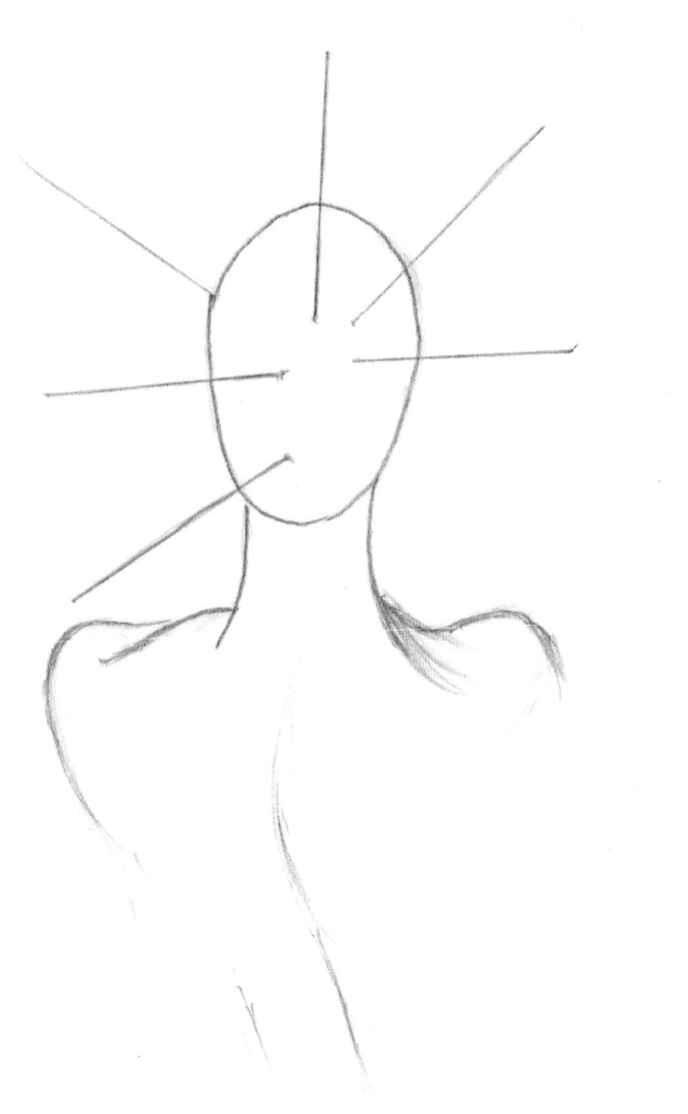

4 April 1998

A jug of steaming, hot water is overturned on my abdomen, and the hot water enters my body. This raises my consciousness to a level that begins with the shades of maroon, after which I reach where there is no sound or vibrations, but only stillness.

27 July 1998

It appears that the *Kundalini* needed to clear my left ear of its blockages. A pulse started to beat on the left side of the head, above the neck, and over the ear. It then shifted into the ear and then the palate. After much pulsating, and reaching the left temple, the breath became smooth.

28 July 1998

Twice, I feel the sharp stab of pain in my right toe. The phase of conversation without registering its content goes on. Consciousness returns, moving over waters which are smooth and shining with little ripples. The movement is peaceful. My awareness is low. It seems as if I move in and out of sleep. I later learn that *Guruji* has hurt his toe and it makes me wonder whether the stab of pain I felt earlier was on account of the shared consciousness between the *Guru* and disciple.

29 July 1998

I find myself moving over dry earth. Then, consciousness goes deep within the spleen on the left side of the abdomen. Going in and coming out, circulating in a free flowing movement, the process goes on for at least ten to fifteen minutes of the meditation time.

30 July 1998

My energy field is being cut from the outside with scissors coming in closer towards the body. I discover that it is *Guruji* who is doing this. This results in my disassembling and dispersing as dull golden balls of different sizes. Probably, the atoms have to be rearranged for further experience to unfold. I lose awareness till I find myself behind the door of a large room, which is full of cribs.

Off and on, when awareness returns, I see myself talking to people, looking at charts and figures. I start travelling over shimmering black waters on my way back, till I reach the land, and then, find myself moving down a sloping road with trees on its sides. Obviously, I have been to another realm where the surgical operation to renew the atoms had to be carried out.

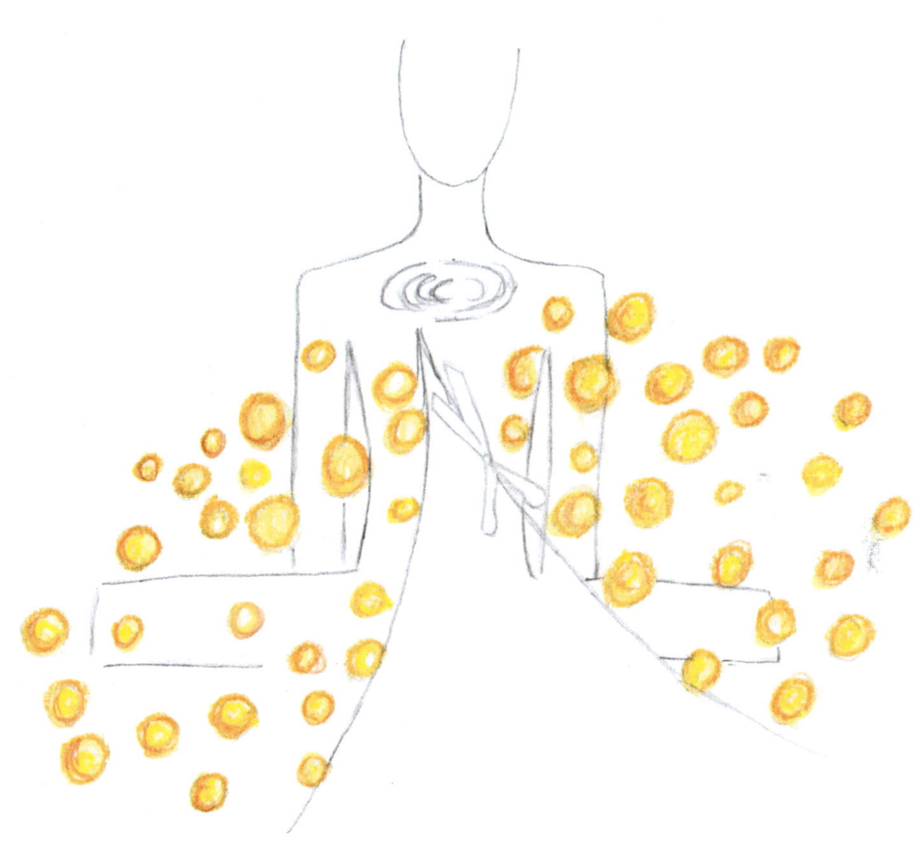

31 July 1998

A hand in the void lets slip a ball, which comes rolling towards me. Midway, it becomes a huge bird, like an eagle, which flies towards my head, heralding in a new wave of consciousness.

1 September 1998

Image gazing. After reading, in Baba Gagangiri's book, about image gazing, I start practicing *tratak* in the early hours of the morning. Nothing much happens, probably because I saw all the different faces I was to see when, on *Guruji's* suggestion, I had practiced gazing at a black circle. However, this further enhanced my focus and concentration.

4 September 1998

My reflection in the mirror starts turning black at the edges.

5 September 1998

The right side of my head and body is fully lit, like the screen of a monitor. Consciousness is like a huge book, the pages of which turn gently on their own, and then go in reverse. There is pain and discomfort in the head because I feel the brain shifting its place. What probably takes place is a shift in consciousness a couple of times. At one stage the chest radiates a white light, and then, golden light.

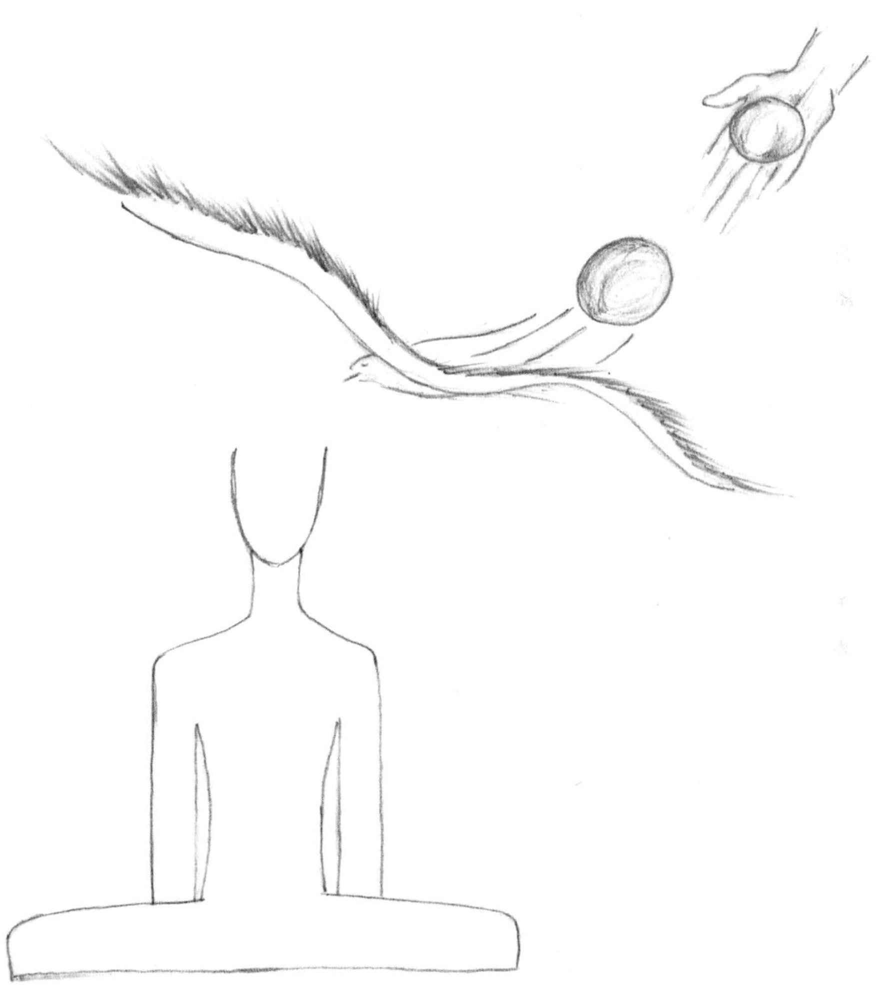

7 September 1998

The left side of my brain extends and, forming a curve, it starts to move towards the right side of the brain which has opened out like a flower. The left brain moves into the deepest region of the right brain, which is filled with white light. Can this be a vivid depiction of the critical-analytical probing of the unconscious mind, which this journey in meditation largely represents?

"If we imagine ourselves looking straight down into the bell of a flower of the convolvulus type, we shall get some idea of the general appearance of a chakra. The stalk of the flower in each springs from a point in the spine, so another view might show the spine as a central stem, from which flowers shoot forth at intervals, showing the opening of their bells at the surface of the etheric body."

– Leadbeater – 'The Chakras: A Monograph', op. cit., pp. 4-5.

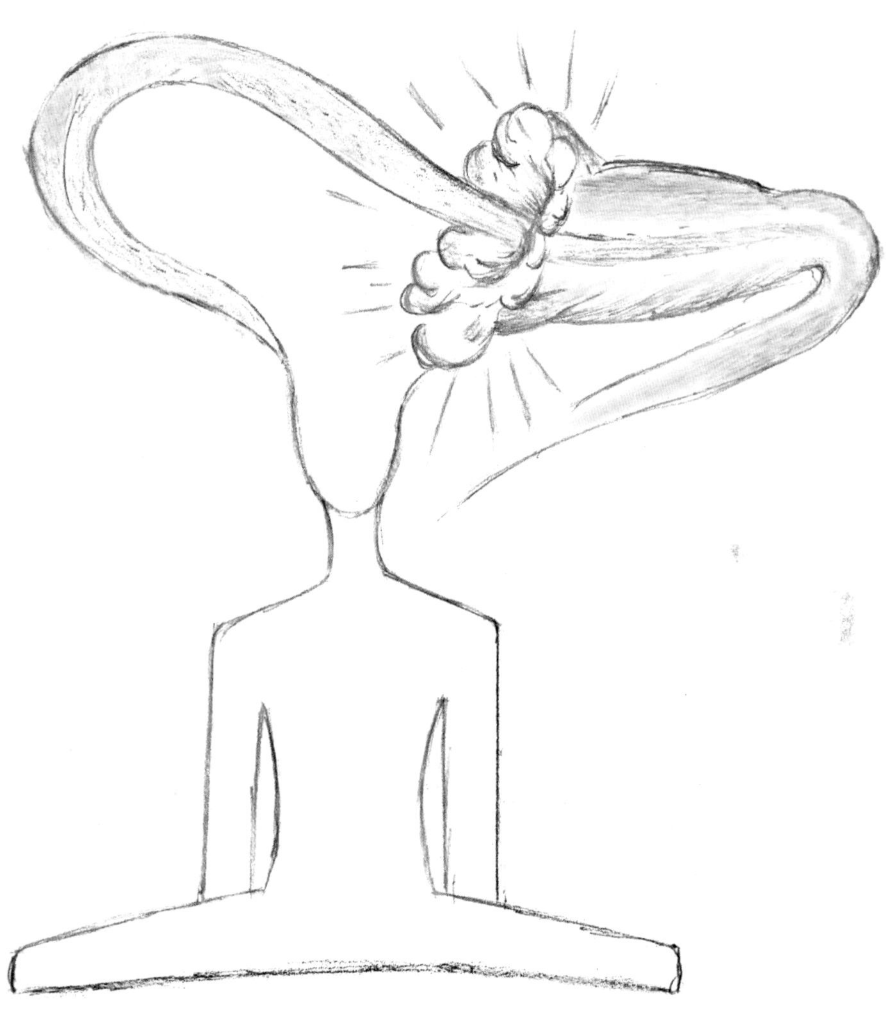

10 September 1998

I am at a golden, egg-shaped, vibrant level. A lump of earth with green grass growing on it is put on my head like a cap.

"This illustration brings clearly before us an interesting fact connected with the yellow light, which signifies intellect. When this color is present in the oval, it invariably shows itself in the upper part of it, in the neighbourhood of the head; consequently it is the origin of the idea of the nimbus or glory round the head of a saint, since this yellow is much the most conspicuous of the colors of the astral body, and the one most easily perceived by anyone who is approaching the verge of clairvoyance. Also, even without astral sight it may occasionally be perceived; for when any person of some development is making a special effort of any kind, as, for example, in preaching or lecturing, the intellectual faculties are in unusual activity, and the yellow glow is therefore intensified."

– Leadbeater, C. W. – 'Man Visible and Invisible'.
The Theosophical Publishing House, Adyar, India, 1925. Eighth Reprint, 1999, pp. 108-109.

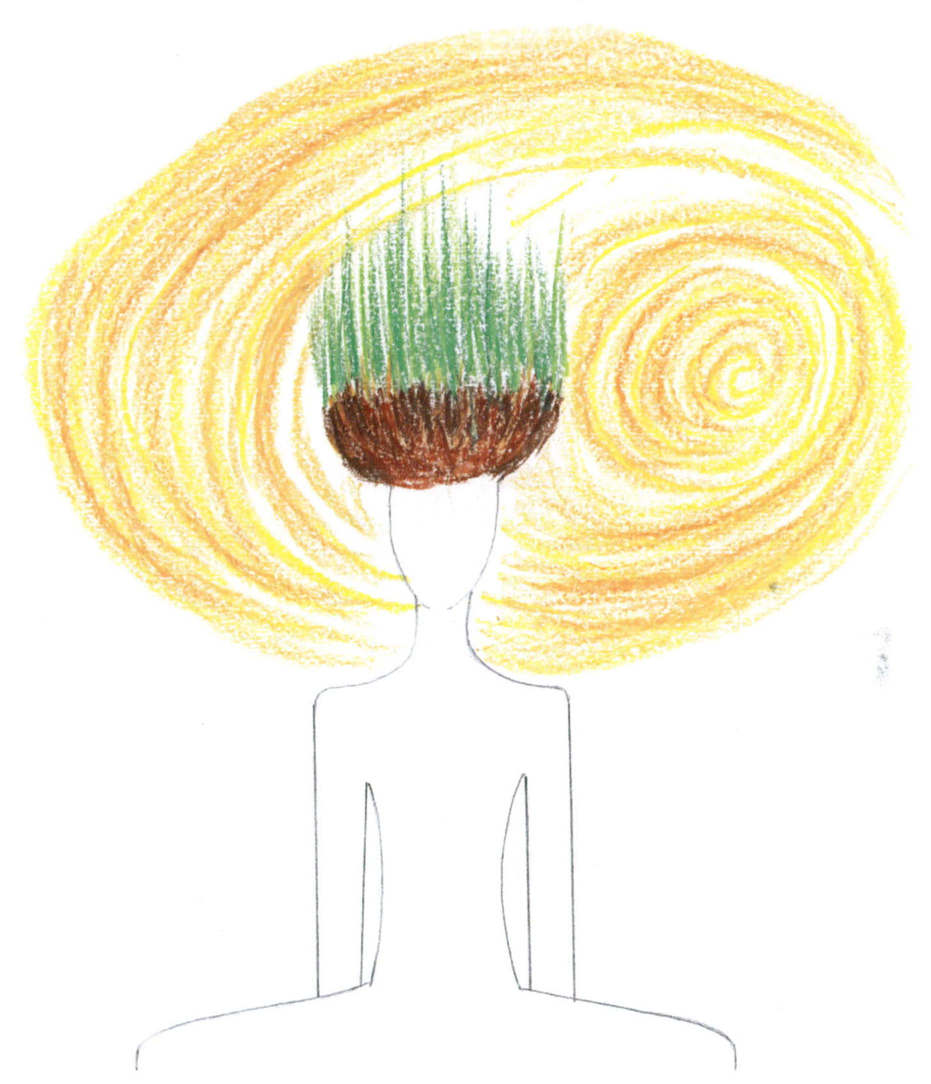

10 September 1998

Then, I see a dagger rising, and blood splatters all over me, as though there is a blood sacrifice. The visions remind me of the rituals for worshipping the Goddess during the *Navratri* festival that is soon to commence, and I wonder if this is another instance of identifying with the Universal Consciousness.

The realisation dawns that what I am being shown is that the Creator, the Created, and the Destroyer are but One.

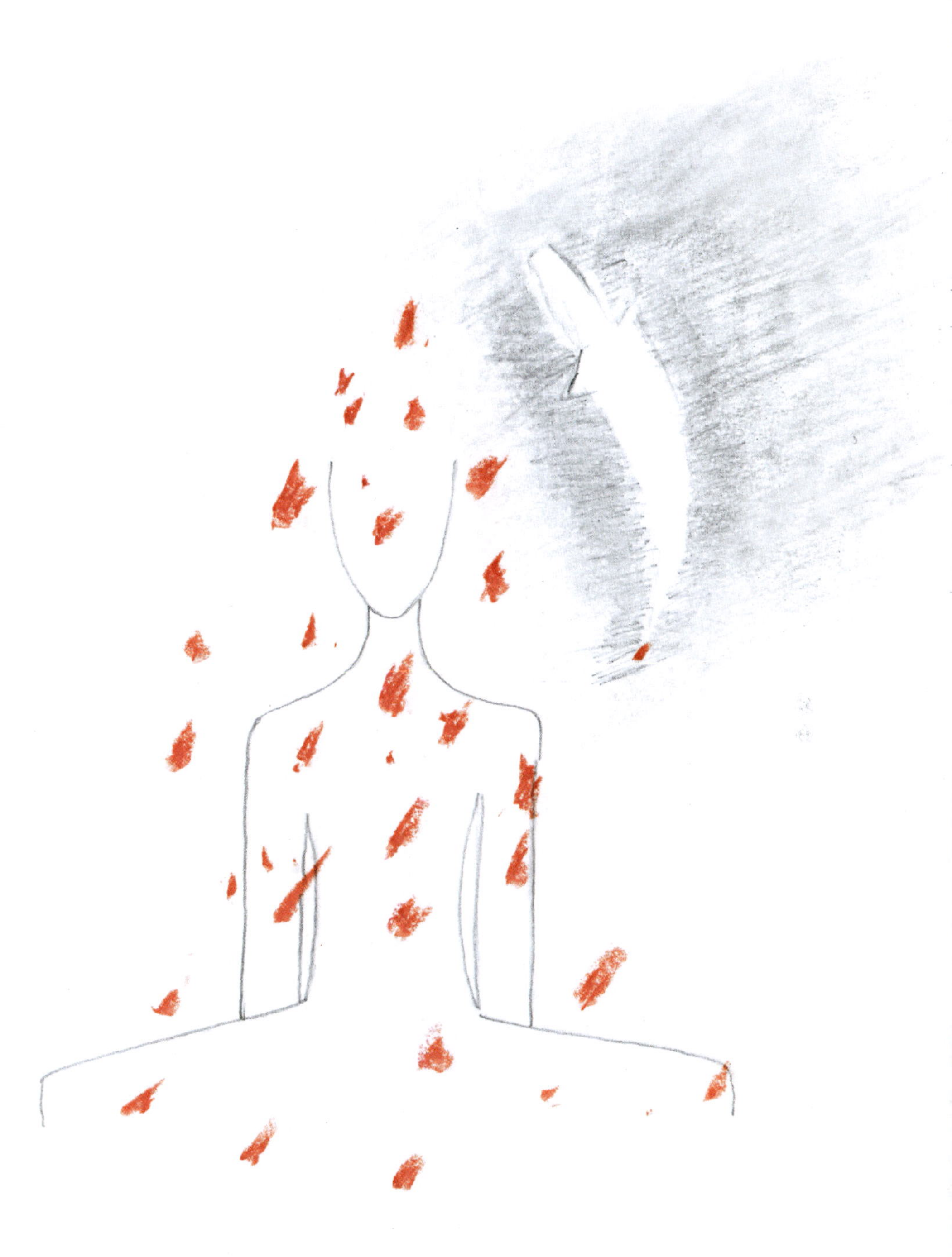

11 September 1998

This time I see the vibratory level as silver. I raise a shield over my head. It has holes in it, through which beams of silver light are poured all over my body, sitting in meditation. The steel sieve is to protect my body and mind from the power of the lightning silver rods. Though this shattering of the residue *karma* was required, the higher self took needful precautions in order not to cause undue damage. There is seen the *Sushumna* as a spear-like rod around which a *chakra,* in the form of a silver disc, rotates.

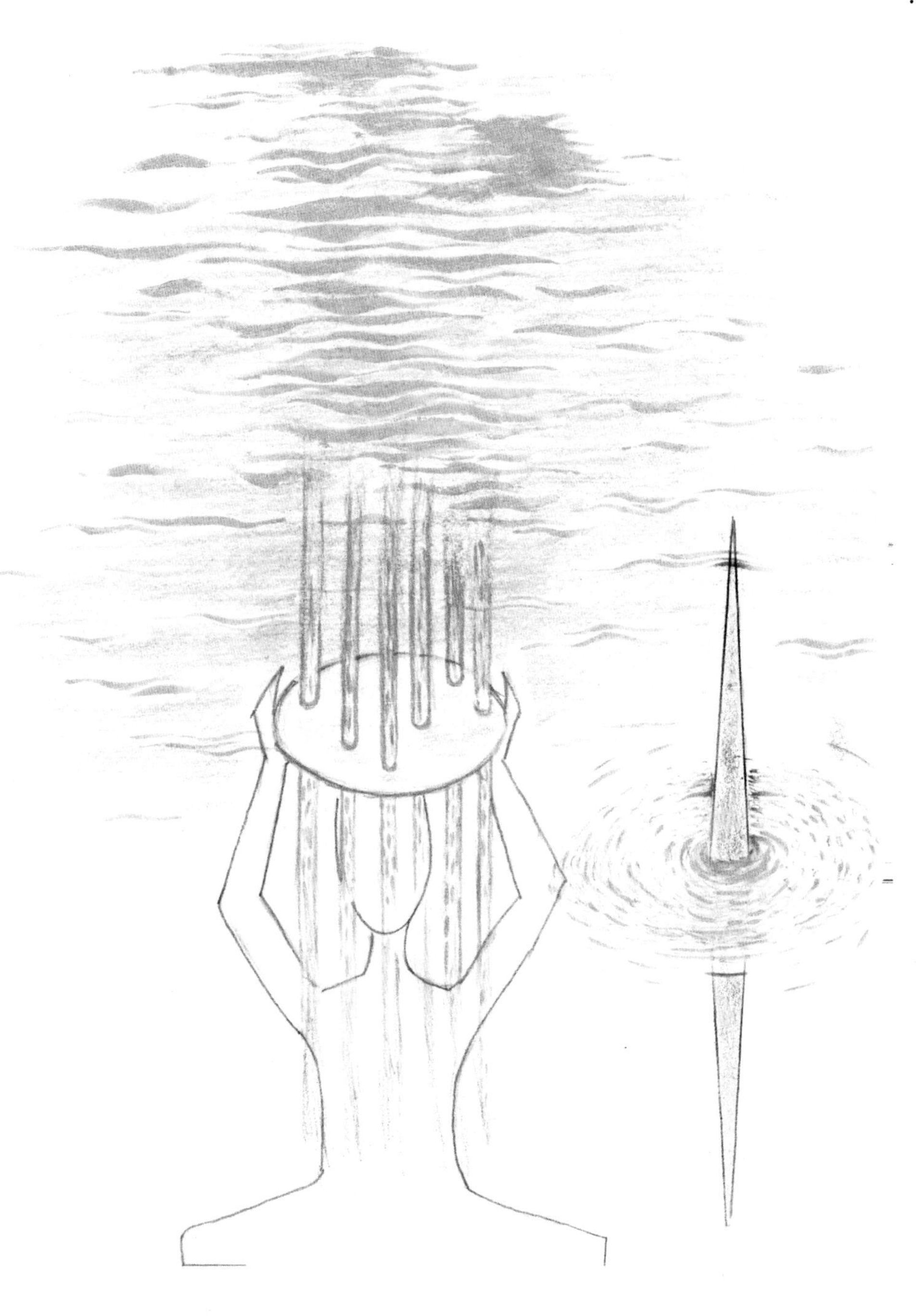

12 September 1998

I see a spoon and a small bowl being readied for something, and wonder if I'll be given something to eat this time. Then, I see the spoon being lifted and something being poured into an opening in the forehead. My body starts to fill up and it expands from the left side, stretching all the way to the right, until the consistency or the density changes and I begin to flow. In order to get back together and return, I start moving in a cone-like fashion, mainly white but with a hint of maroon, until I reach a certain gravitational level. Then, I find myself flowing as a mass of gray.

18 September 1998

The session begins with a shift and a drop in the left brain, more like an aircraft losing pressure or altitude. The body moves out of the scene and spreads in different directions. At some stage I am asked whether I want to continue, or some such thing. I say, "might as well go all the way." At times, I find myself holding my head and my consciousness starting to identify with different aspects of nature. I am a bird, and I sense another presence. I see a raven take off and follow me. Suddenly, I am like a cross and I move in a vertical direction, at a great speed, through a vibratory level that seems to be like yellow butter in colour and consistency, until I reach the silver level. I then start to come back as a silver rod rotating anti-clockwise. I feel some pressure or a sensation at the back of the skull, off-centre, towards the top. I hear someone calling me "Charolette."

It seems that the body-mind intellect has been given time for it to adjust to the changes wrought by the descending energy in the form of silver rods, before the ascending energy starts to rise from the base of the body very purposefully. A shield, like the one I was holding over my head, is now on my shoulders, probably to control the flow of energy as it moves towards the head. This complete purification was probably being done for a big revelation. I await its unfoldment.

This shielding seems very necessary, as otherwise, such massive doses of energy could just blow me up or reduce my nervous system to cinders.

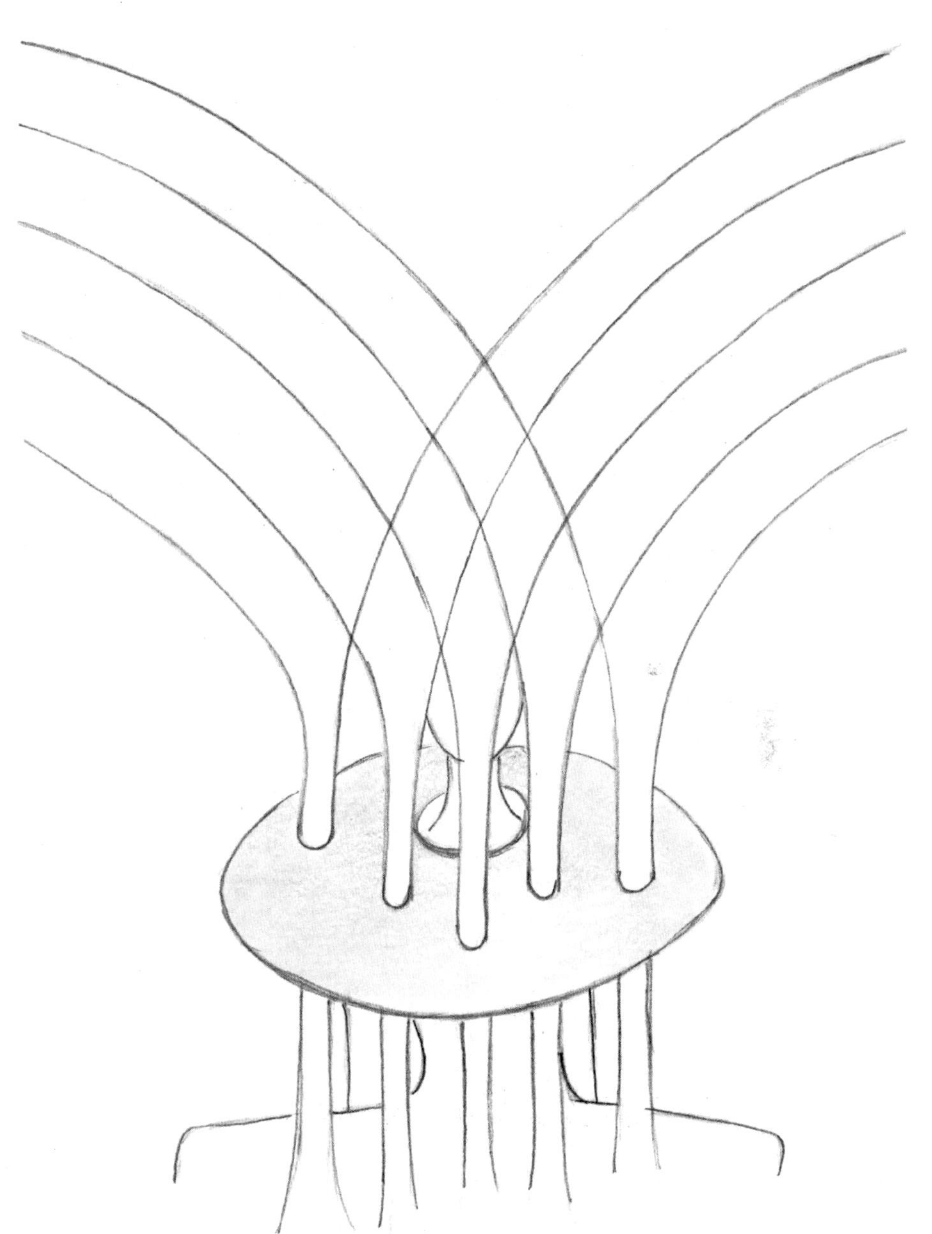

19 September 1998

A young and healthy-looking Doberman Pinscher dog with a shining coat comes to me. Whenever I see a dog, I intuitively identify it as the energy field of *Lord Dattatreya*. The whole meditation session seems different, somehow. I feel heaviness in my body, especially in my feet. The energy starts moving and, as it moves, the body becomes a shining golden snake. Its mouth opens wider and wider as it moves upwards and simultaneously turns into itself, leaving a *Shivalinga* of light placed in its head. This completes the process of purification for my body-mind organism.

"...and the third in sahasrara chakra (paralingam). It is said that in sahasrara chakra the finest consciousness resides in the shape of an illuminated shivalingam."
– Muktibodhananda, op. cit., pp. 533-534.

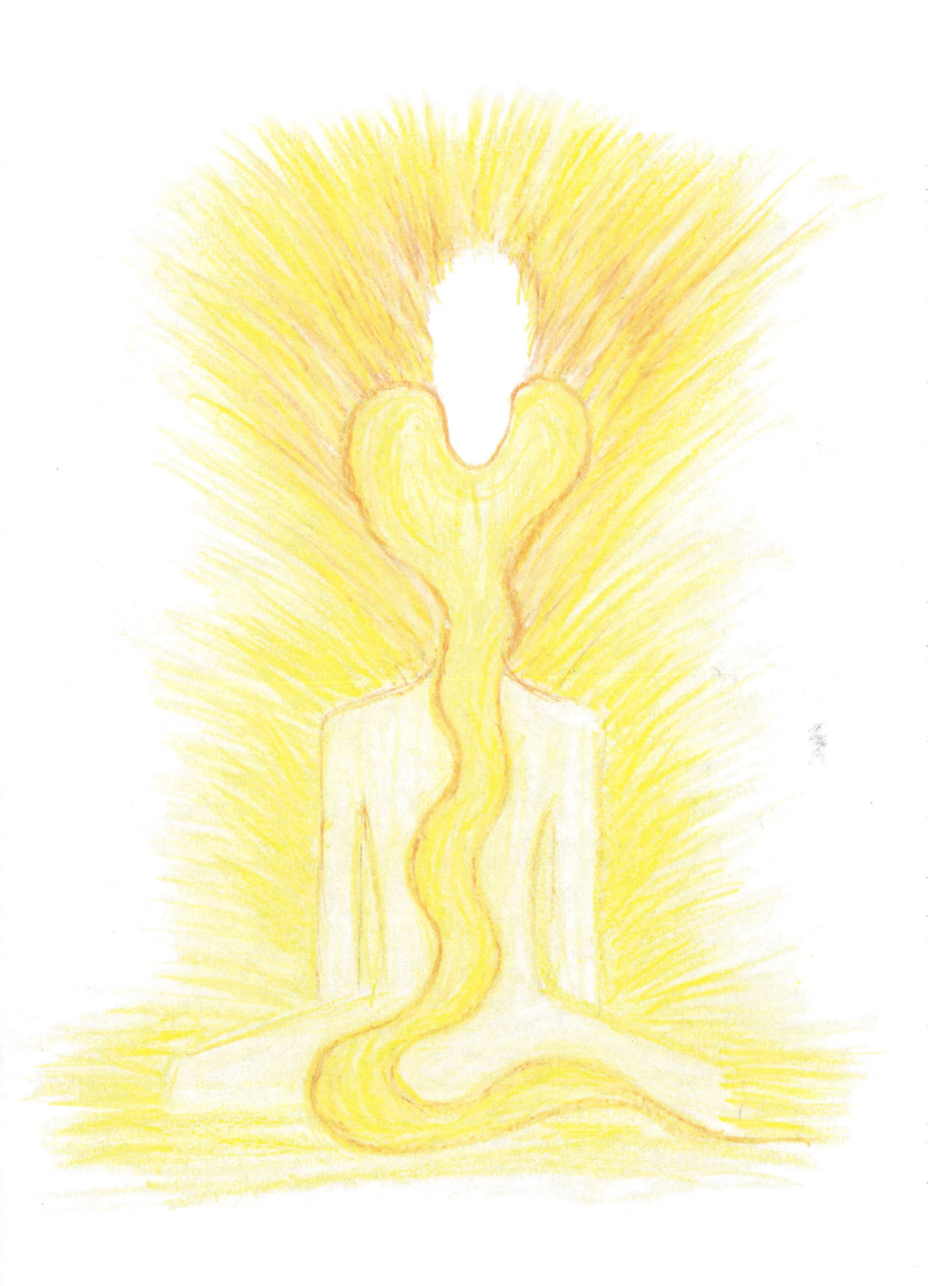

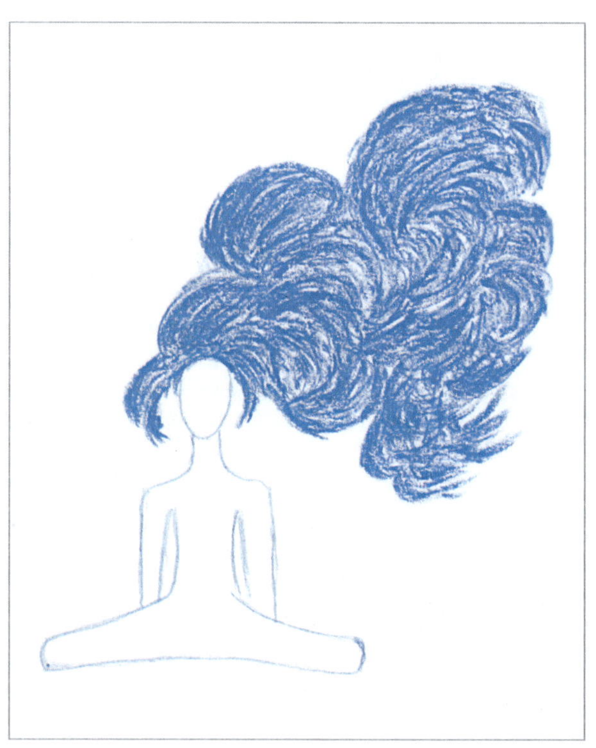

PSYCHIC ATTACKS

The psychic attacks during the course of unfoldment of my spiritual dimensions have made me realise the person I have been or am, in the physical dimension. I took all psychic attacks with equanimity, probably because I was always focused in the moment. There was no data, script, or dialogue prepared for the event, because there was no preconceived expectation of any untoward happening, with the result, I delivered what the moment demanded. Invariably, the appropriate action was taken with full awareness and in a precise manner. I realise now that this was a reflection of the person I am in my physical day-to-day life. It was the balance in my physical, emotional, and mental dimensions which made the equanimity possible. Since there was no preconceived data, the attacks were watched and experienced with a sense of curiosity, wonder, and adventure. The understanding dawned that though the attacks seemed very forceful and physical, no physical pain was felt. This was because the attacks were from the subtle dimensions and could impact only my subtle dimension i.e. my psyche. Anyone with a weaker nervous system would probably be left with some sort of aberration. One requires presence of mind and nerves of steel to stay present and in the moment when undergoing a psychic attack.

Psychic attacks vary in their presentation. Some are experienced at the physical level, while others at the mental and emotional levels. Given below are some of the psychic attacks at different levels of consciousness:

a. Being attacked and molested. I turn as wrathful as *Kali* and bite off the attacker's tongue and spit it out with vehemence.
b. Another time, a practicing *tantrik* is attacking me. I respond by throwing myself in the air and spinning at top speed; I fling myself at the *tantrik,* and shatter him with a sound like a loud clap of lightning.
c. Then, there is another *tantrik* who, with his fixed, piercing gaze, beckons me; I just look back at him with normal gaze.

d. At another time, I felt as if I was physically and forcefully flung from my bed. This gave me the biggest shock. It was so real, I had to switch on the light and figure out what happened.
e. Suddenly, during meditation, as if out of nowhere, gnome-like figures appear in different sizes and shapes. Some are grotesque, while some have peculiar twists to their facial features. Their main purpose is to frighten the daylights out of you. If you don't get scared with their pranks, they can start pulling at your hair and ears, and climb on to your shoulders.
f. If all this does not work out, they start playing with you. They will shower you with kisses, get behind you and shut your eyes. As long as you ignore them and are playful when required, they are quite harmless. It can be quite entertaining to observe.

If you are going through these type of experiences, rest assured that if you can go through them without reacting and maintain your balance, you might even enjoy them. They are like any challenge you face in life.

Chapter Five

THE KEY TO CREATION

The *Ajna* and *Swadhisthan chakra* move in unison to give me further knowledge.

"Ajna is the bridge which links the guru with the disciples. It represents the level at which it is possible for direct mind to mind communication to take place between two people. It is in this chakra that communication with the external guru, teacher or preceptor takes place. And it is here that the directions of the inner guru are heard in the deepest state of meditation."

– *Saraswati, op. cit., p. 129.*

"Swadhisthana is regarded as the substratum or basis of individual human existence. Its counterpart in the brain is the unconscious mind and it is the storehouse of mental impressions or samskaras. It is said that all the karmas, the past lives, the previous experiences, the greater dimension of the human personality that is unconscious, can be symbolized by Swadhisthana chakra."

– *Saraswati, ibid., p. 148.*

The brain, body, and the mind having been worked upon, it seems that I am ready for the *Guru* to lead me on to a higher level of consciousness.

29 September 1998

Group meditation: The energy is very concentrated. I can see the energy going around *Guruji*, encircling him and then coming back towards all of us who are sitting for meditation. The whole room fills up with silver energy.

"This form was generated by one who was trying, while sitting in meditation, to fill his mind with an aspiration to enfold all mankind in order to draw them upward toward the high ideal which shone so clearly before his eyes. Therefore it is that the form which he produces seems to rush out from him, to curve round upon itself, and to return to its base."

– Besant, Annie & Leadbeater, C. W. – 'Thought Forms'. The Theosophical Publishing House, Adyar, India, 1925. Tenth Reprint, 1992, pp. 57-58.

Whenever I find that my head is becoming heavy and congested with energy during meditation, I take *Guruji's* hands and place them on my head. This invariably dissipates the energy, or perhaps the *Guru* absorbs it.

30 September 1998

Early morning: I experience a very deep meditation. The *Ajna chakra* extends endlessly in front, causing pressure in my left brain. It reverts to its position, and then the *chakra* in the right temple moves clockwise at first, and then anti-clockwise. Consciousness is at first focused in the centre, and later, moves upwards from the *Ajna chakra* and out of the Crown *chakra*. The entire process is repeated. The energy is free flowing. It feels as though the consciousness has gone somewhere, returned, and assimilated what the left brain has brought.

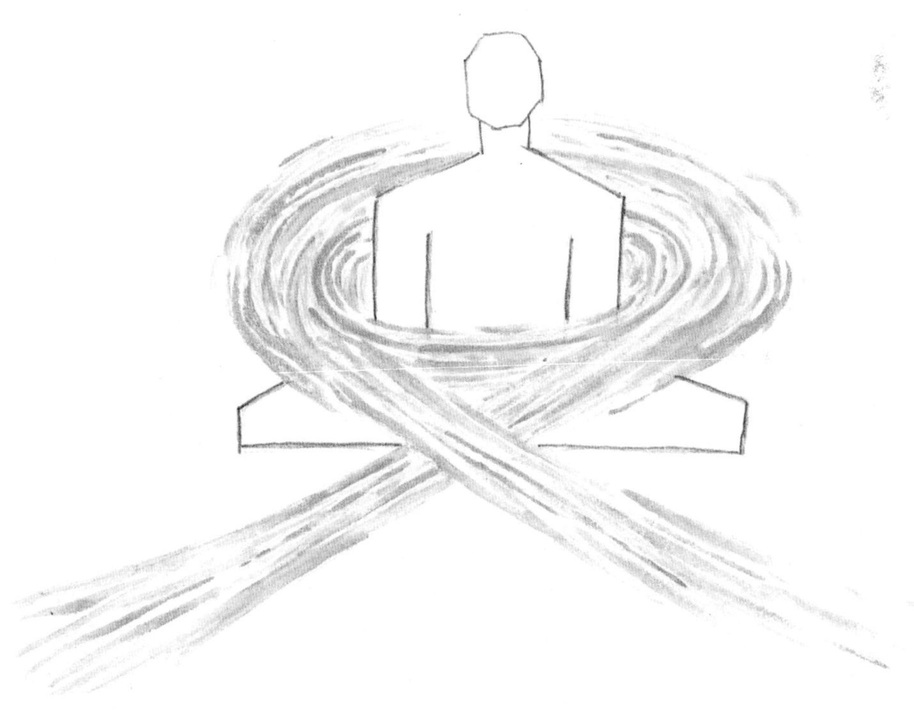

30 September 1998

8:30 am: If not immediately penned down, one loses the thread or sequence of the thought process. The energy moves freely and then I think it becomes denser, or perhaps it is passing through a *nadi* which is not too clear. The fragrance is exotic. In front of the forehead, I can see a crocodile with its jaws opening and shutting. The vibrations of the *Swadhisthan chakra* seem to have moved up to the *Ajna chakra*. The vibrations are felt more acutely in the right side of the brain; the *chakra* seems to be opening and closing. The movement of the energy in the head is constrained. It starts clearing and I see myself over gray clouds. I suddenly see myself as a translucent, green bird flitting across the blue sky, and then I am in the void. I sense concentrated pain in the top right side of the brain. The pain must be quite sharp, for I think of *Guruji* and speak to the *Kundalini,* asking her to be gentle. I try to relax, and manage to last out the entire process until a centre is somehow activated, so that I sense myself as being upside down in my own head. I feel the vibrations of the *chakra,* and see them as my legs opening and closing in my head. I have not been able to figure out what this detailed visual is supposed to tell me.

> R. A.: The crocodile could be a dramatic representation of the reptilian brain being forced to relinquish its instinctive control, as the mind has evolved considerably beyond mere instinctual control. It is naturally an occasion for pain, as the reptilian brain is very old, very tough, and very enduring, and it does not like being shunted out of dominance. The soaring green bird is a clear symbol of freedom and represents the flight from the mud. It is quite a fight between the old sections of the brain and the sections that are coming into being, which may account for Santosh's inability to decipher the experience.

2 October 1998

4:30 am: I am a part of a field. The plantation is green and it moves gently in the breeze. It has two or three assorted types of leaves, all rather small in size.

7:30 am: I feel and see my left arm (not the gross arm) move in the motion of bending and stretching. I am shown the musculature of the arm without its skin sheath. What is odd is that the arm grows out of my forehead. I realise that the motion of the *chakra,* which is a little off-centre and towards the left, creates the vibrations which give rise to the vision of the arm. I wonder whether I am being asked to exercise and develop my analytical faculties, located in the left brain, for the purpose of this book.

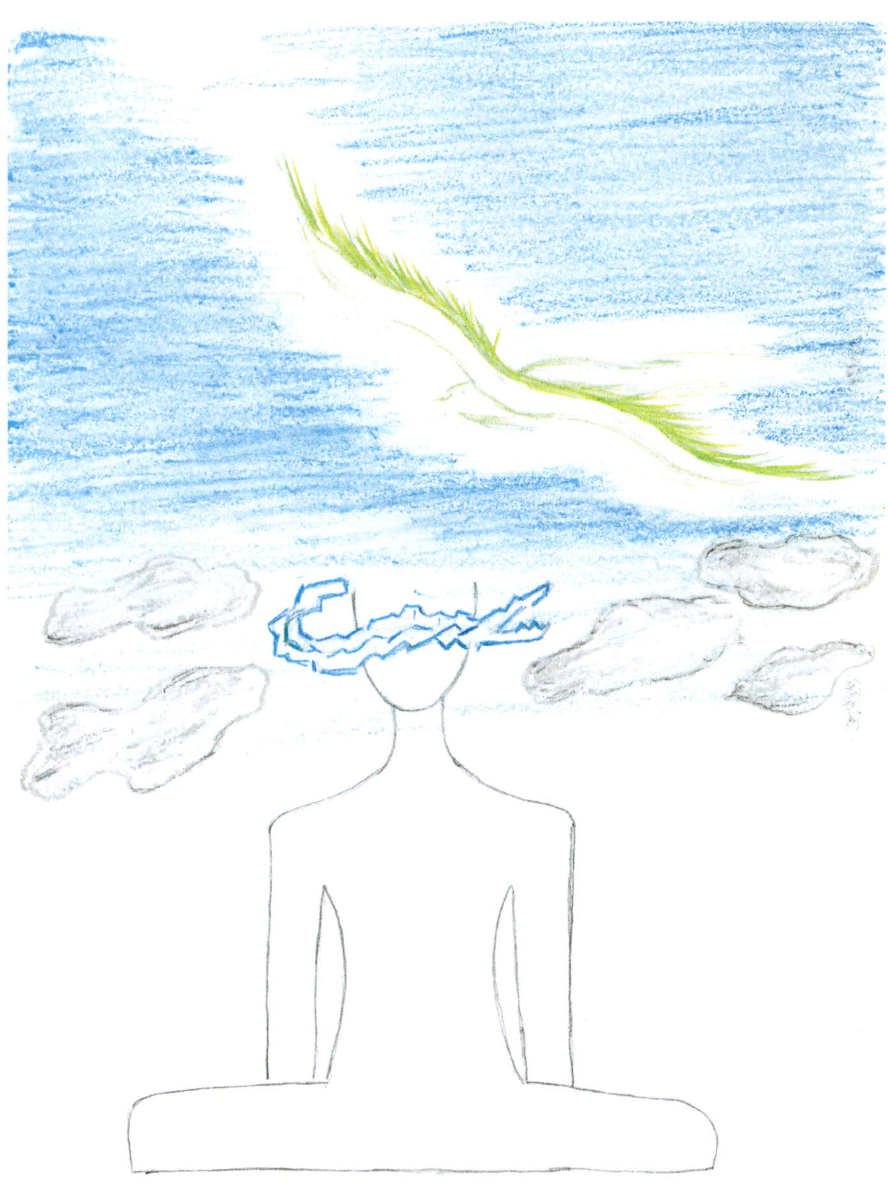

2 October 1998

The *chakra* in the left temple and the *Spleen chakra* seem to be connected. They remind me of the spinning wheel. Both are rotating, until only the spleen seems to be acted upon. I vividly see my spleen being shattered and broken into bits and pieces with a chisel made of light, and then reconstructed. I feel pain in the tips of the left toes. I have not come across much reading material on the *Spleen chakra,* but for me it comes into focus every now and then and many of my experiences seem to be associated with it and its activation.

"The spleen chakra is not indicated in the Indian books; its place is taken by a centre called the Svadhishthana, situated in the neighbourhood of the generative organs."

– Leadbeater – 'The Chakras: A Monograph', op. cit., p. 7.

"The spleen, is devoted to the specialization, subdivision and dispersion of the vitality which comes to us from the sun. That vitality is poured out again from it in six horizontal streams, the seventh variety being drawn into the hub of the wheel... Each of the six divisions of the wheel shows predominantly the colour of one of the forms of the vital force – red, orange, yellow, green, blue and violet."

– Leadbeater, ibid., p. 12.

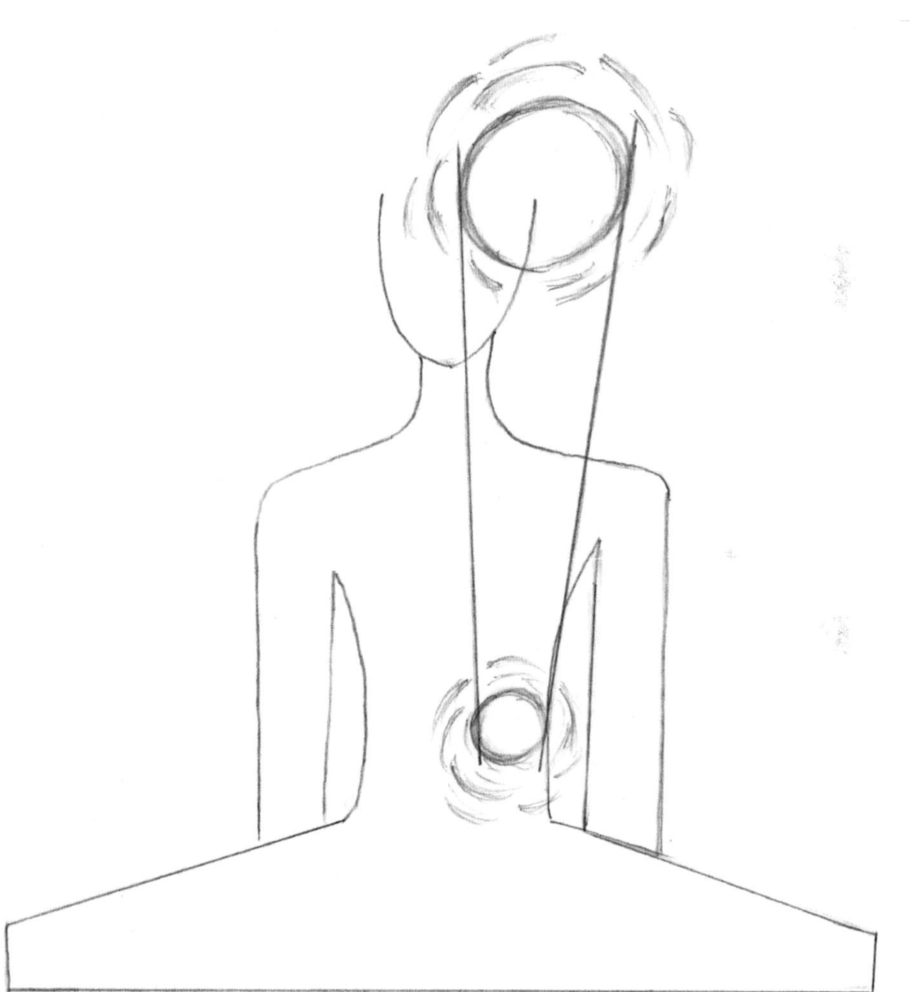

3 October 1998

Meditation is all light. Someone places a gold coin in my hand and asks me to keep it. There is a shift in the vibrations and in the head. My inside resounds with the sound of *Alakh Niranjan*. I start moving through a golden tunnel. Again, there are shifts in the vibrations. These shifts are like vibrations going over a small row of speed breakers. I come to a level where I see and bow down to the golden forms of Buddha and other sages.

"Naths are Aghoris. They make everything in their being self-identify with Lord Shiva even under the most trying and tempting circumstances. Their motto is 'Alak Niranjan'; Alak means 'a-laksha', 'free from attribution or discrimination'. Nir-anjana means 'completely clean', free of any fault, stain or blemish. What is that thing which is undefined and undefiled? The absolute imperishable Brahman."

– *Svoboda, op. cit., pp. 209-210.*

4 October 1998

The energy is concentrated in the right side of the chest; it, in turn, creates a gentle pressure in the brain, above the neck and behind the ear.

5 October 1998

I am moving as a river of silver liquid in a light blue sky. For the rest of the meditation, I am fixed in white light.

6 October 1998

The top of the spine, I am told, and also shown, is known as the wheel. I am what looks like a white steed with huge wings, which are moving in slow motion over my chest. The horse then becomes a big bird like a hawk. I take off after flapping the wings for a while. Throughout the meditation, there is a shift in the scalp, off and on. With the shift, the whole body opens up in two. My flight is slow and the wings seem heavy. Maybe I am not used to this vibratory level yet. At times, I am wholly aware of the silver thread.

11 October 1998

I see my legs criss-crossing at different angles; they are protruding from my head; they turn into two beams of light in motion crossing each other like the 20th Century Fox symbol. Then, once again, the legs take the place of beams. Simultaneously, I see an arm with only the muscular pattern flexing itself. I express that I still don't understand this peculiar vision, which keeps repeating itself.

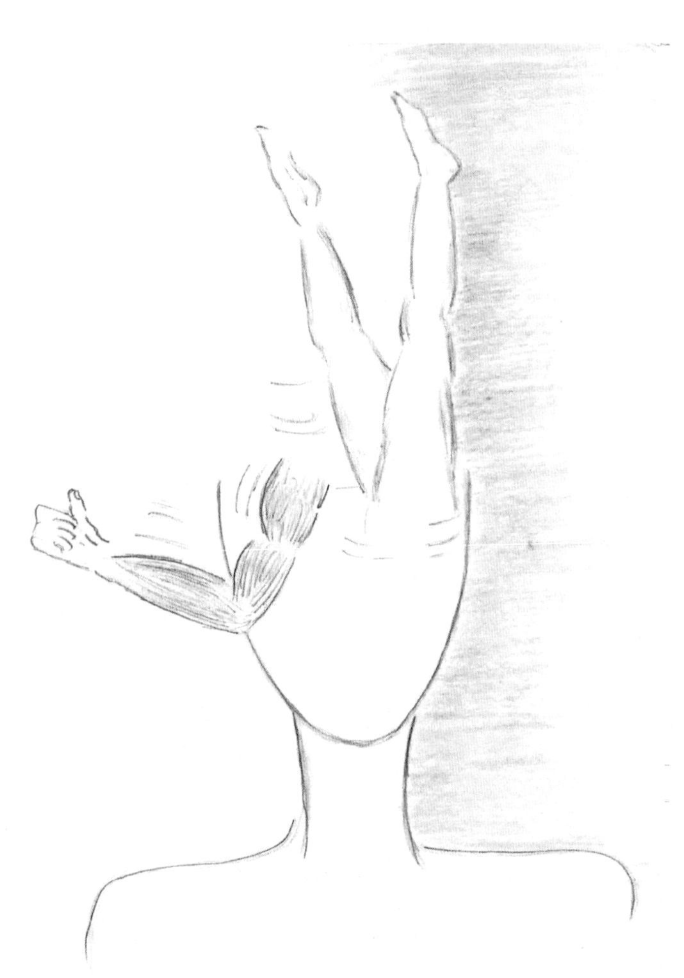

12 October 1998

A vision emerges from the void in front of my forehead. I see a baby-pink breast which fills the sky, with soft, white tufts all over, almost like nimbus clouds. At its centre is what looks like a nipple, with water sprinkling out of it. This vision stays until I acknowledge that I have registered it. Then, across the void appears a huge white lily. I am sitting on its petal in the meditation posture. I raise the question, "What is this?" The answer I receive is, "*Yoni.*" The image of the lily dissolves and I see the whole cosmos begin to move in a pulsating, rhythmic motion of attraction and repulsion, contraction and expansion. I understand this as a deeply moving lesson in the principle of Creation, which on the biological plane would be termed as the male-female union. I now understand the vision of the flexing arm and the cris-crossing legs.

I have drawn most of the visuals as mirror images. Although reversed, the above experience makes me believe that the ultimate symbol of ॐ and the *nada* sound emanated at this vibratory level, with the bindu being represented by the pink belly and the cosmic navel. I realise that I am not even 'this'. I am 'that' which is observing the process of creation.

"In the process of self-realization the highest goal, identified with the arousal of Kundalini, is recognized as a microcosmic version of the feminine power of Sakti. The tantrikas identify the power of Sakti with Cosmic Consciousness, since she projects the biunity of male and female principles... In surrendering we become feminine, the feminine depths of our psyche then dissolving, transcending – a total experience of oneness – and a tremendous energy is released... The state of ananda, of infinite joy or perpetual bliss, is reached. This state of bliss is the closest approximation one may experience to the state of liberation. The inner life-force is aroused to its full potential through the mystic process of awakening the Kundalini Sakti... This crucial experience is one of the great moments of our spiritual existence."

– Mookerjee, Ajit – 'Kundalini: The Arousal of the Inner Energy'. Thames and Hudson Ltd., London, 1982. Reprinted, 1995. pp. 59-63.

"In its state of perfection, of total awareness
It is unaware of its awareness;
then consciousness stirs into a moan of Aum,
and the dream – creation – begins.
It is conscious of being,
It exults in this beingness.
Immersed in the love of I-am-ness,
It expresses itself in duality."

– Balsekar, Ramesh – 'The Whole Truth'. May 1979, p. 3

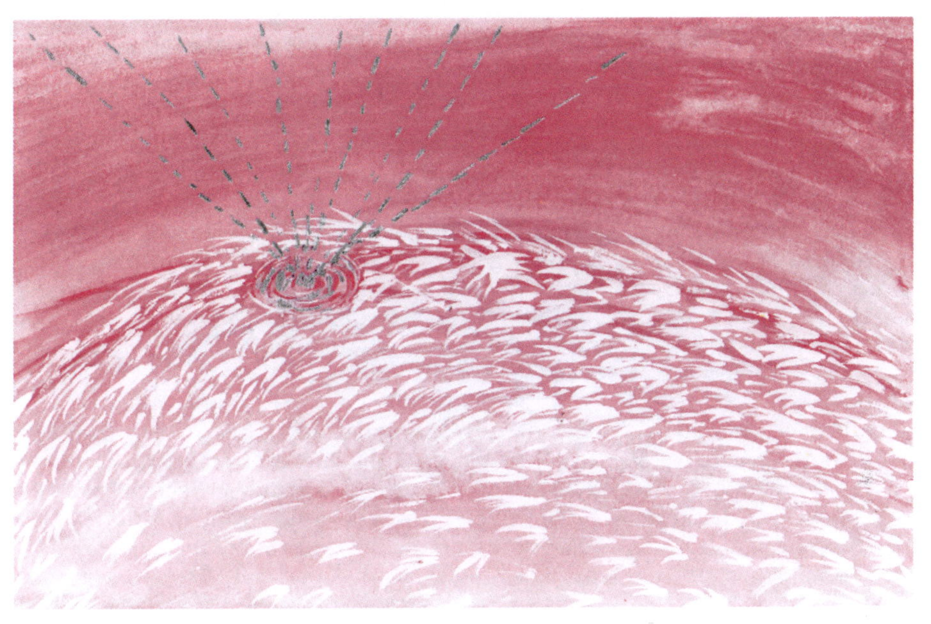

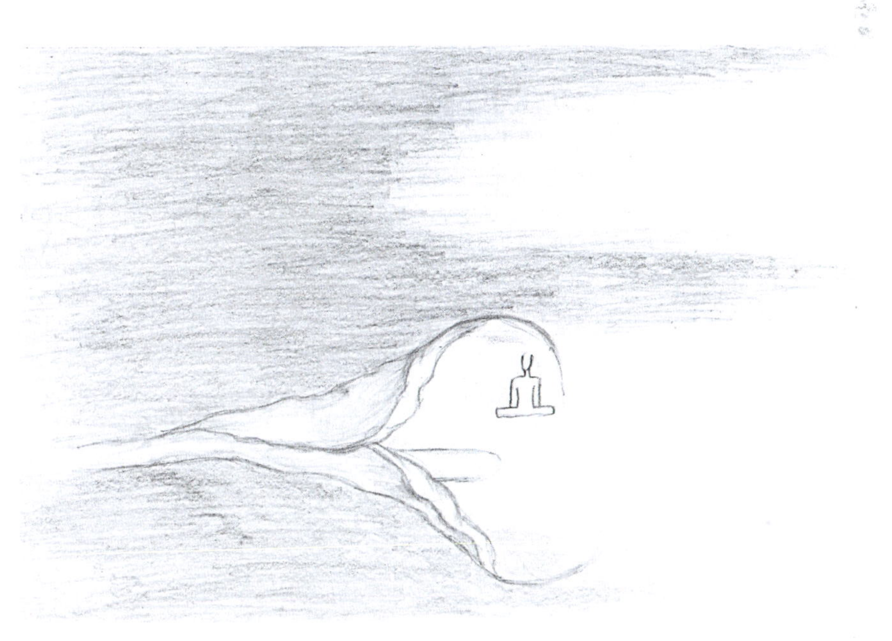

17 October 1998

7:30 am: I see *Guruji* coming towards me. He tells me to get into some sort of vehicle that he is driving. At first, we circle in a clockwise direction over shimmering black water, and then we take off, reaching a level where there are only white flames flickering. At some stage in the meditation, I see a beautiful snake sitting on my chest and looking into my eyes, and then it sinks into my chest, followed by *Ganpati.*

Realisation dawns that every gross manifestation has its duplicate in the subtle realm. Whatever takes place in the physical realm has already first taken place in the subtle realm. There is a lag time, which I have not been able to determine. Perhaps it varies from one event to another. As I understand, the whole creation is duplication of form from one species to another – an insect can look like a twig, another one can look like a leaf, a fish can look like a butterfly or a carrot. The same patterns are repeated in the multitude of Creation.

20 October 1998

The vibrations start rolling towards me like a coiled spring (Fig. 1). As they come closer, I see that they are like deep waves coming at a certain speed, giving the effect of a rolling spring (Fig. 2).

23 October 1998

After the spring-like vibrations, meditation seems to have stabilised, in the sense that consciousness seems to be moving in a slow and gentle motion. I get occasional glimpses of past and perhaps future events.

Fig. 1

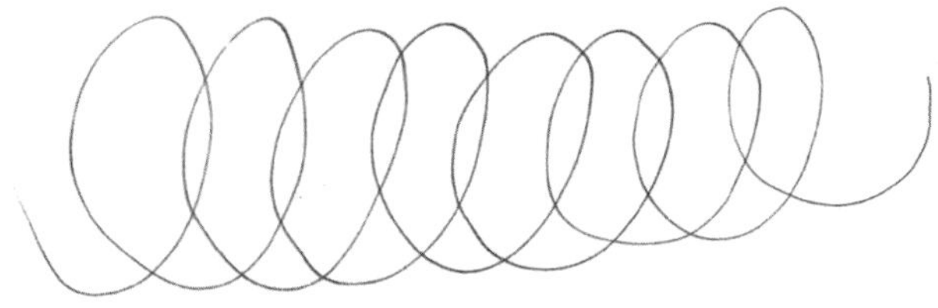

Fig. 2

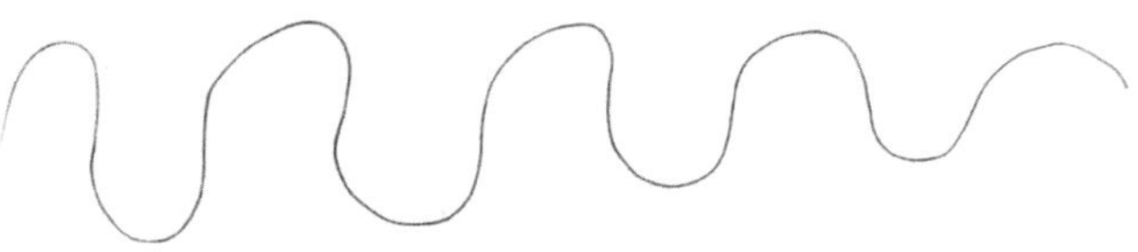

2 November 1998

Ever since I started watching the breath, and that is not very long ago, I found that it has no fixed rhythm or pattern. It can fluctuate according to the state of the mind or vice-versa unless, of course, the mind is completely relaxed or there is no mind. I realise that the breath is the vehicle of the *Prana*, the life force, and is also the vehicle of consciousness. Wherever the breath goes, consciousness is there in the body. Watching its movement makes me also aware as to where it is free flowing, and where at other places it is having to force or manoeuvre its way around.

2 November 1998

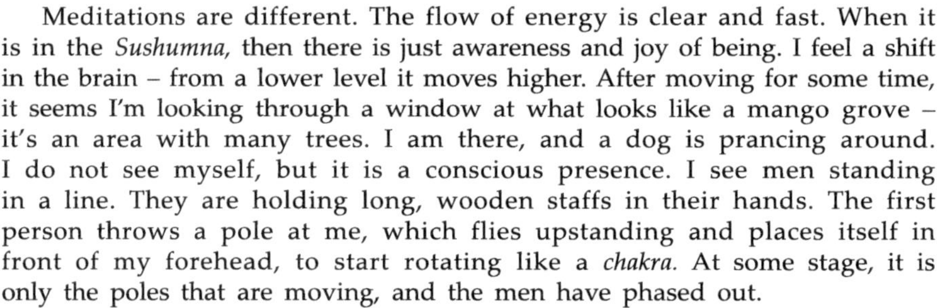

Meditations are different. The flow of energy is clear and fast. When it is in the *Sushumna*, then there is just awareness and joy of being. I feel a shift in the brain – from a lower level it moves higher. After moving for some time, it seems I'm looking through a window at what looks like a mango grove – it's an area with many trees. I am there, and a dog is prancing around. I do not see myself, but it is a conscious presence. I see men standing in a line. They are holding long, wooden staffs in their hands. The first person throws a pole at me, which flies upstanding and places itself in front of my forehead, to start rotating like a *chakra*. At some stage, it is only the poles that are moving, and the men have phased out.

As soon as the left brain starts to work, I become aware of the energy starting its smooth journey again. My breathing has shifted to the navel. I come to huge, golden gates, which leads me to think, "At last, I'm done with the last couple of rickety gates encountered in earlier meditations." I look forward to what this new experience will bring. I am breathing through both the nostrils. I sense a large figure standing with arms spread out wide. Somehow, I think of Osho. He seems to embrace me as emptiness, with myself looking on as Consciousness. At this level, no vibrations are felt, and only the *Prana* is felt. There are no landscapes or anything identifiable – there is no day or night, no light or dark, no heat or cold – it just IS!

"Nothing is more real than nothing." – *Samuel Beckett*

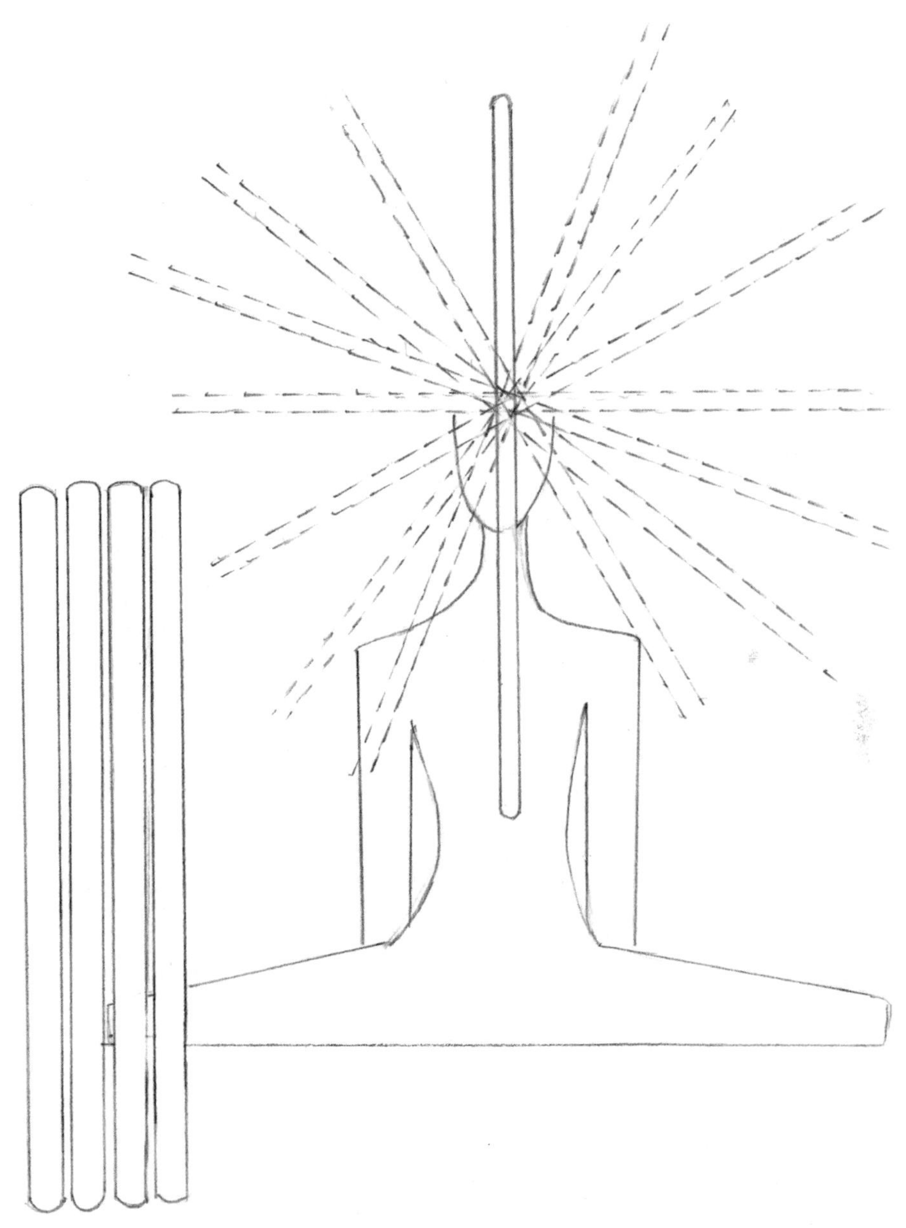

4 November 1998

While I sit in meditation there is a feeling of light, and a vibration in the form of a spiral comes and places itself in between my eyebrows. It gently starts pushing my consciousness backwards till I feel I am becoming smaller and smaller. The spiral is a dull, flaming red in colour. The pressure continues till consciousness takes a turn and I lose awareness.

6 November 1998

4 am: While meditating, there is a sensation on the left side of the head, a little above the neck, as if a drill is being pushed into the skull. The vibration reminds me of the dentist's drill.

7 November 1998

The right brain comes towards the left brain and creates a barrier.

I start the recitation of the affirmations and notice that it becomes all garbled. The words are not forming. The breathing seems to have stopped.

13 November 1998

I see myself as an African woman. I roll out of my body and when I stand up, I am tall and well proportioned, wearing a long dress and a flowing headgear.

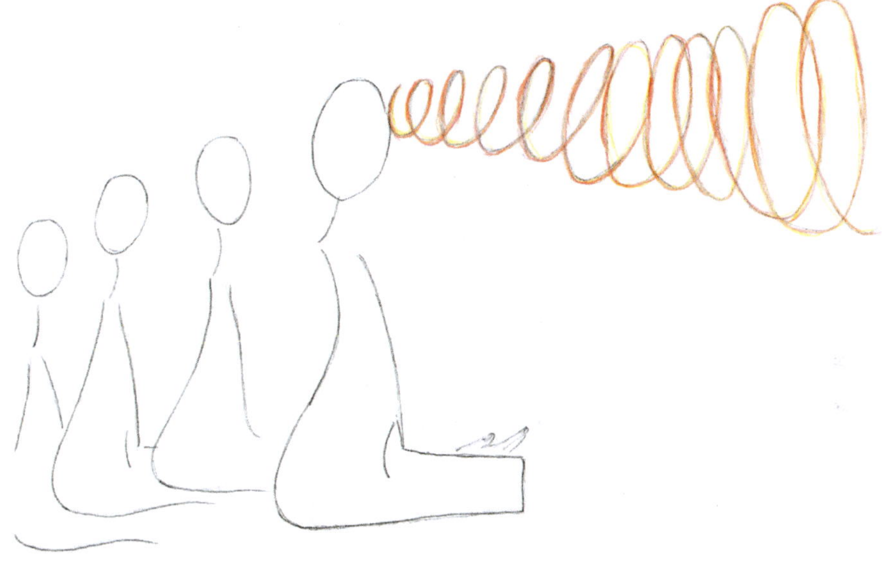

14 November 1998

The meditation is significantly different. A finger places itself on my forehead between the eyebrows (*Ajna chakra*) and starts putting pressure till all affirmations are stopped. I feel the head within my head turning like a revolving door. The adjustment is somewhat stressful. I also find the body within trying to move in the same manner. The *chakra* at the back of the head starts to get active, bringing about a smoother functioning of the whole process. I see a man's face talking to me; it is a face from another planet – the features are like ours but the shape of the face is slightly different. The main difference is in the ears and the jaw. The jaw has a problem forming the words. Am I supposed to learn something? I don't know if I did! My head is still slightly heavy.

16 November 1998

The *Ajna chakra* and the *Muladhar chakra* move simultaneously clockwise and anti-clockwise – one at the top and the other at the bottom, supported by a long hub. I suppose at the subtle level, this is all the structure that we have. The dense body forms around it.

23 November 1998

The Heart *chakra* in the etheric body seems like a cartwheel. It is first rotating fast and smooth in a flat fashion, then turns at an angle, like a dish-antenna rotating at the same speed.

It then starts to move on its edge and shifts into the centre of the body and chest in a sawing motion.

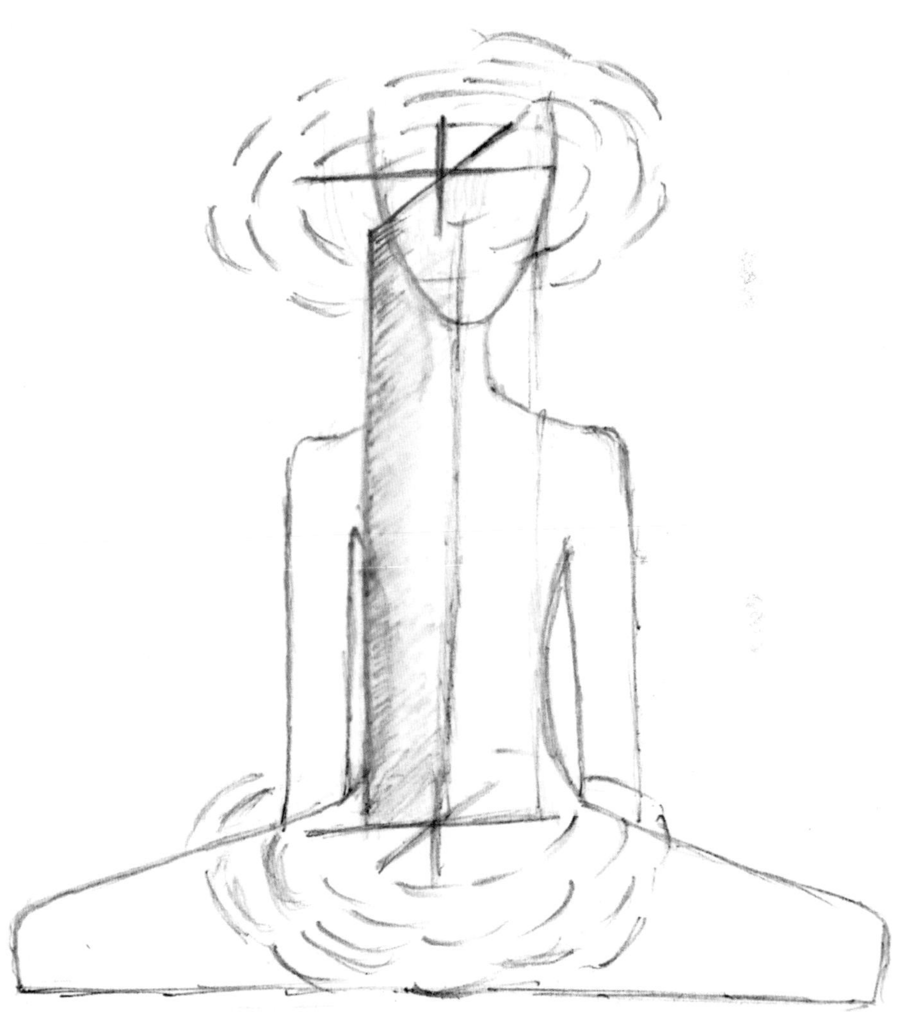

27 November 1998

I see myself at the end of a long, silver thread hanging like a drop. In due course, I disengage from the thread and plonk! I fall into the ocean creating ripples. This marks the merging of the Individual Consciousness with the Cosmic Consciousness.

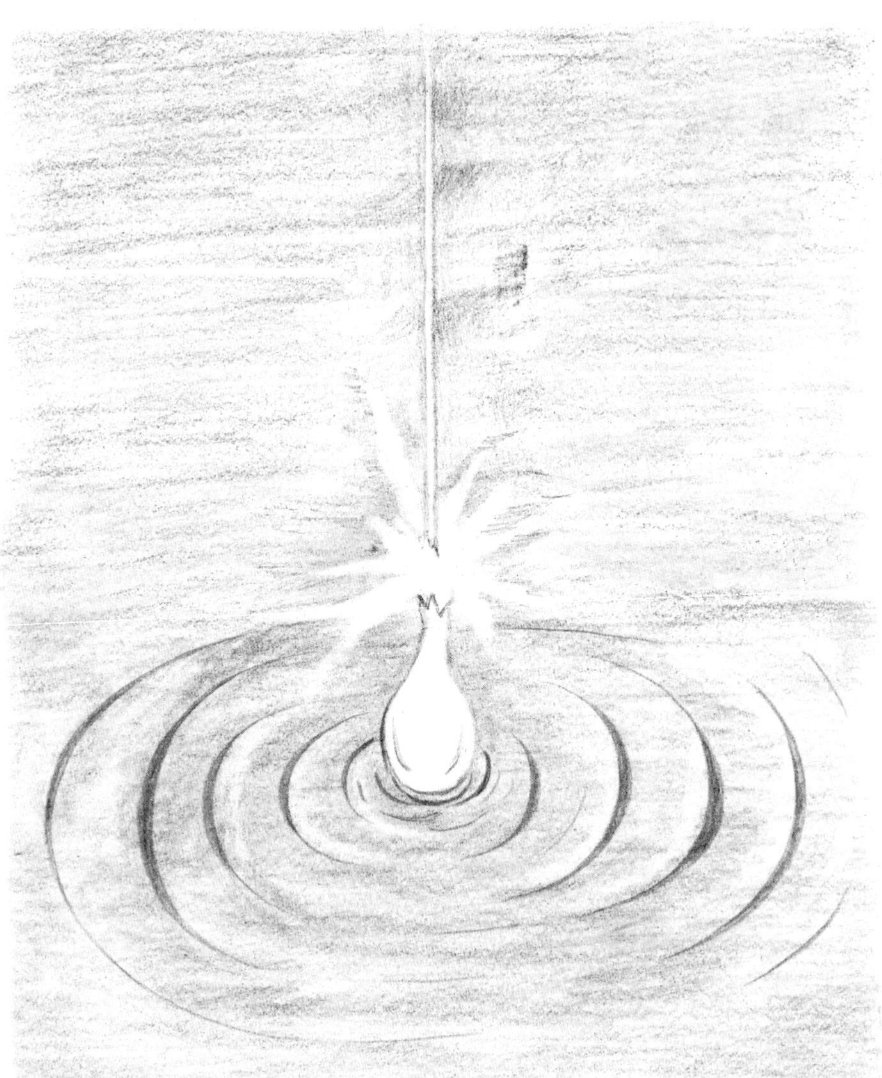

1 December 1998

Outside the right temple, the *chakra* seems to have taken the form of a screw-driver and is moving in line with my vision, straight into space. After some time, it shifts into the head, slowly moving into the left brain at an angle. The right temple is shining with shimmering light on the outside. There is a click in the right brain, and consciousness shifts to another vibratory level. The shift is very smooth.

It seems that the Individual Consciousness has to dip deep into the Cosmic Consciousness to come back renewed and, having re-established a contact with the Whole, for further knowledge to unfold and lend clarity to my understanding of the origin of my Source.

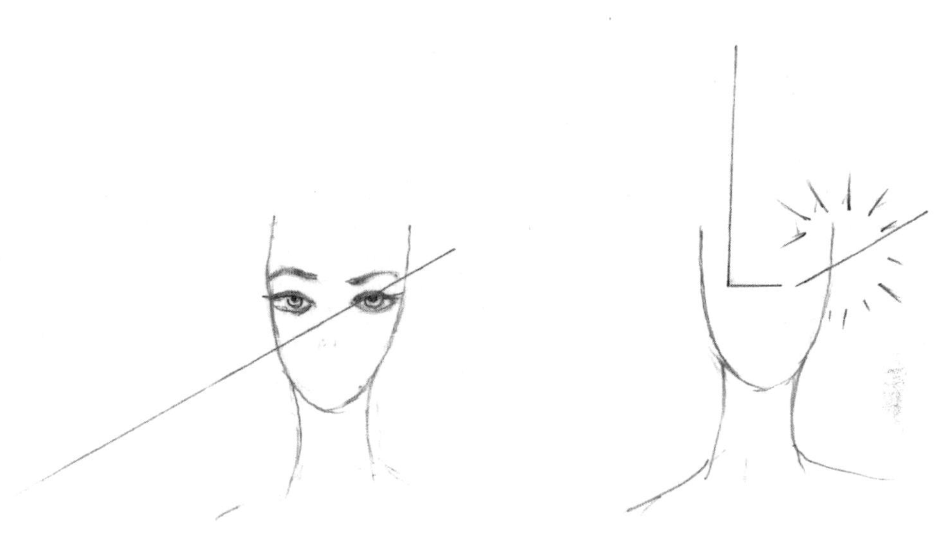

7 December 1998

A beam of white light starts from a point at the back of the head, near about where the neck and head meet, it projects itself out, curves over the head like a big cobra hood and, still curving over the front of the body, enters the chest. Simultaneously, another beam of light projects from the same point and shoots up like an antenna into the cosmos.

This point at the base of the head (which was activated with acupuncture earlier) would now serve for me as the connecting point or as the service station between the Individual Consciousness and Source Consciousness. It is awe inspiring to know that I am now directly connected with the Source. Wow!!!

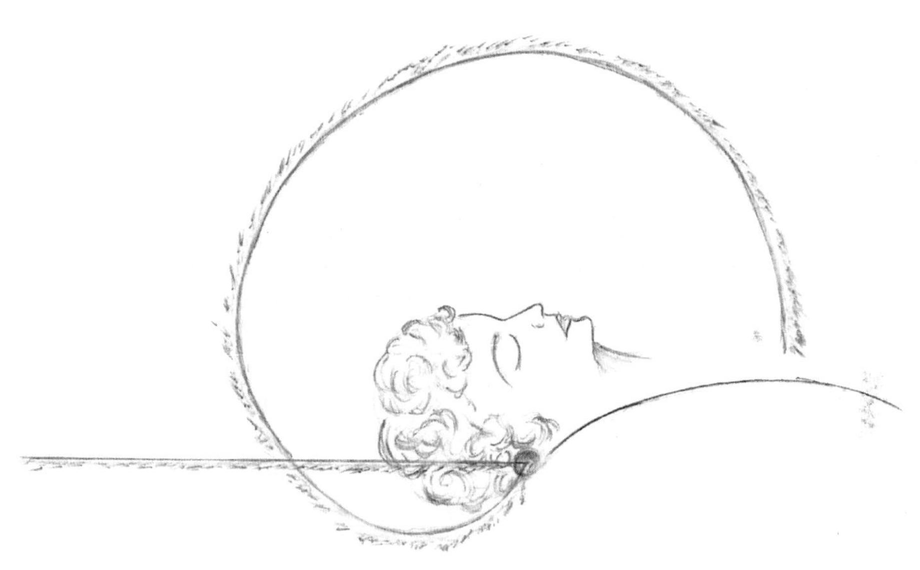

8 December 1998

Group meditation: I see a huge *chakra* in the form of a gigantic wheel rotating above us. Consciousness emanating from the *Guru's Ajna chakra* moves out and towards the group and encompasses all of us.

9 December 1998

Since two days, there is a sensation of all the cells vibrating to a particular type of rhythm.

I see a burning yellow, red, and golden cocoon. A tiny black snake glides into it and the pulsating and rhythmic movement of the cosmos within itself starts all over again. Is it the womb and the sperm? Am I watching the process of creation manifesting from the subtle into the dense form? The zigzag pattern I have drawn, *Guruji* says, is the DNA.

> *"Bindu is both macrocosmic and microcosmic. Ultimately there is maha bindu (the entire conscious creation), then para bindu (the form of Ishwara), sukshma bindu (the individual mind) and sthula bindu (the gross bindu in the form of ovum/sperm). The emergence of bindu is the evolution of the primordial Shakti into manifestation of mind and matter."*
>
> – *Muktibodhananda, op. cit., p. 464.*

I am full of gratitude to the grace of the *Guru*, Source, *Kundalini*, the Invisible Masters, and Spiritual Guides, who made it possible for me to go through this experience in total awareness, and also gave the ability to function at the abstract level of knowing and understanding. It must be my good *karma* coming to the fore.

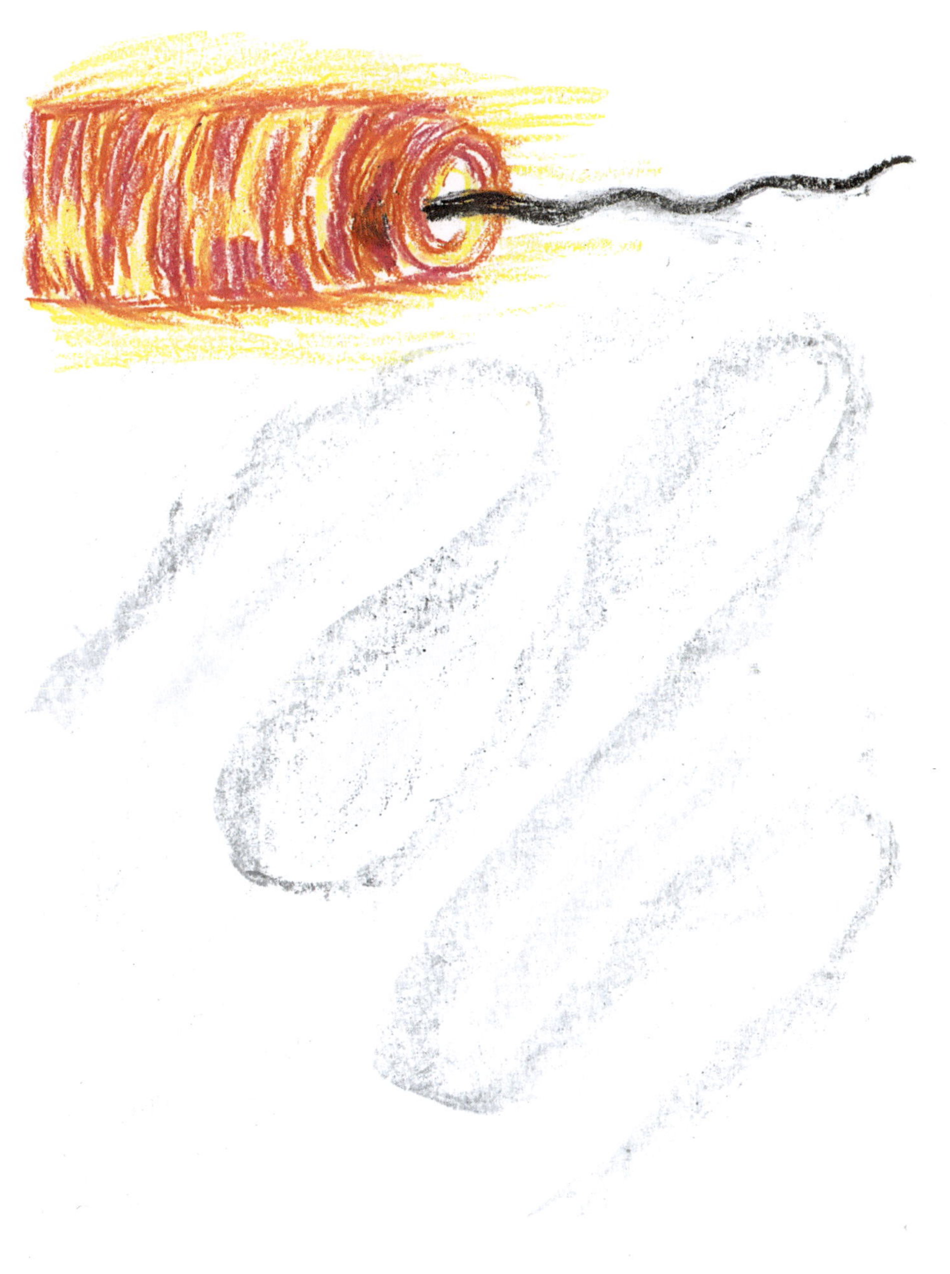

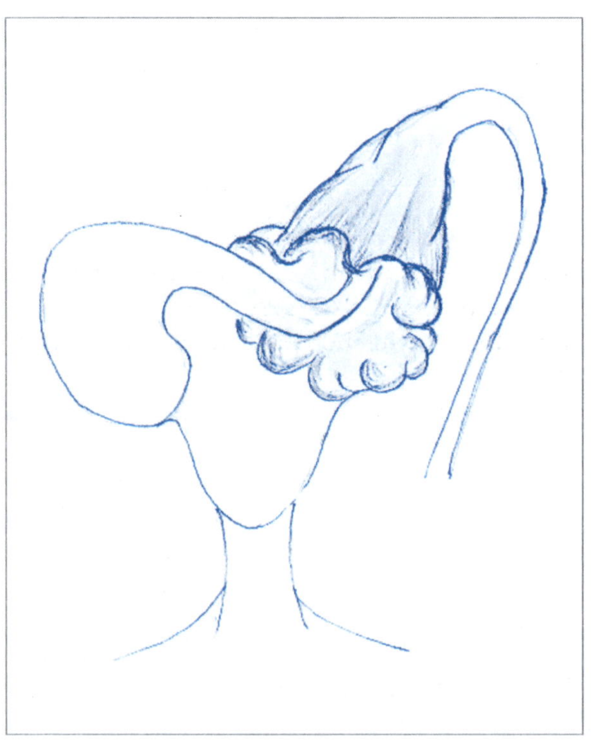

SHIFTS

As an individual grows from childhood, to youth, to adulthood, and so forth, a natural and a gradual shift takes place in his consciousness of which he is totally unaware. It is a smooth transition from one level to the other. The brain structure and grooves develop accordingly. It is a constant development that goes on as adjustment to his/her life situations occur.

However, if one is following a programme in self-development, the process is different, particularly if one is following *"Kundalini yoga."* The only way for an aspirant to go through this *yoga* is to have full faith in the *Guru,* a complete surrender to the energy, and the knowledge that whatever his/her body-mind intellect is made to go through is only for its good.

As I followed the path of *Kundalini yoga,* I realised that my salvation lay in surrendering to the energy and fearlessly leaving myself open to its working. The clearing of my mental, emotional, and physical blocks was hastened by the awakened *Kundalini,* which meant that the solidified blocks would have to be chiseled and dissolved for the energy to make any headway. This would naturally cause pain and discomfort, shoves and nudges, jerks and twinges, because the energy that is moving is all powerful and will not have any obstacles in its path. The meridians in the subtle body are not expanded enough to take on the extra load, and hence, go into a spasm when the energy moves, which is reflected in the physical body as jerks. One can imagine the immensity of the power that lies dormant within us at the base of the spine when one realises that it is the same energy that causes an earthquake when it moves under the surface of the earth.

I feel I am one of the lucky ones, for I quite enjoyed the experience inspite of the pain and the popping and shattering sounds along with regulating and adjusting the *chakras* that seemed to have got stuck or rusted, for lack of proper functioning and harmony in my body-mind intellect. It was more of an adventure, probably because it was a journey into the unknown. A journey that had no milestones or warning signs. The child in me was most curious to follow the visual experience through; taking in her stride whatever obstacles came along and seeing what this all was leading to. I became apprehensive when the work on the brain started, for this was no child's play. It was serious business. Could I leave my psyche open to any short circuits that might take place? Could I risk going mad? These are the few questions that came to my mind. Could I risk my sanity for the thrill of adventure and excitement thereof? After much thought, I resumed my practice safe and secure in the knowledge that if so far I had been dealt with gentleness, love, and understanding, there was no reason it would be otherwise, at this crucial juncture.

After consideration and reviewing my faith in myself and in the gentle force, *Kundalini* once again started its work like any master craftsman, minutely and efficiently. In order to make it easy for me, I was given full understanding of what was being done in my brain. For me, the shifts that would probably take lifetimes were being cut short by actual manoeuvring of portions of the brain from one centre to another; certain areas were made to move from the left brain into the right brain. Certain parts of the brain had to be stretched by inserting a sharp instrument into the tissue or membrane. Then, the grooves of the frontal lobe had to be erased and re-inscribed. The whole exercise is painful and can take days, depending on an individual's level of tolerance.

I had to go through the process of transformation in order to have my desire to know my source fulfilled. I realise how important it is to be conscious and aware of each thought we have or express because, in doing so, we set the whole body structure in motion to produce the result.

So no more expressing thoughts, wishes, and desires at random, because you have no idea of what you are doing to yourself!

Chapter Six

DEATH OF A BODY AND BIRTH OF A SOUL

"In India, ajna chakra is called divya chakshu (the divine eye), jnana chakshu or jnana netra (the eye of knowledge) because it is the channel through which the spiritual aspirant receives revelation and insight into the underlying nature of existence. It is also called 'the eye of Shiva'."
– *Saraswati – 'Kundalini Tantra', op. cit., p. 130.*

Swami Satyananda Saraswati tells us that "the relationship between *Guru* and disciple is the most ultimate of relationship; it is neither a religious nor a legal relationship. *Guru* and disciple live like an object and its shadows."

What I notice is that the *Guru's* grace is constantly flowing towards all of us. How many of us awaken and get on to the bandwagon depends entirely on our receptivity, willingness to trust, surrender, and our level of evolution.

15 December 1998

Today during meditation I saw that we were all sitting on the *karmic* wheel that was earlier above us, with the *Guru* as the central figure controlling it. Collective Consciousness starts to flow towards the *Guru,* merging with him, and moving out again. Earlier, I recognise him as my *Guru* on my *karmic* wheel and now I see him as the *Guru* of the multitude.

> R. A.: This is practically a *thanka* with the *Guru* in the central space and the lesser lights arranged round the spokes and rims of the cosmic wheel. This vision gives an idea as to why the artists used to make these gorgeous circular diagrams; that was how they experienced the visions of the deities and *Gurus* that crowd the Tibetan faith.

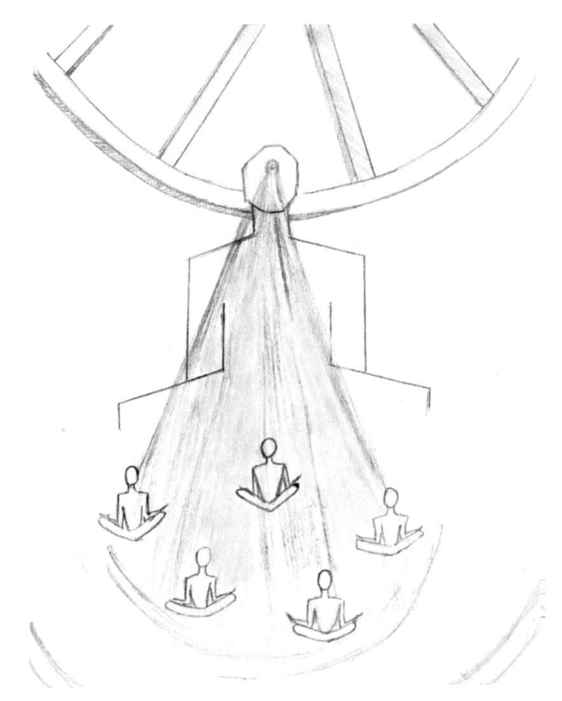

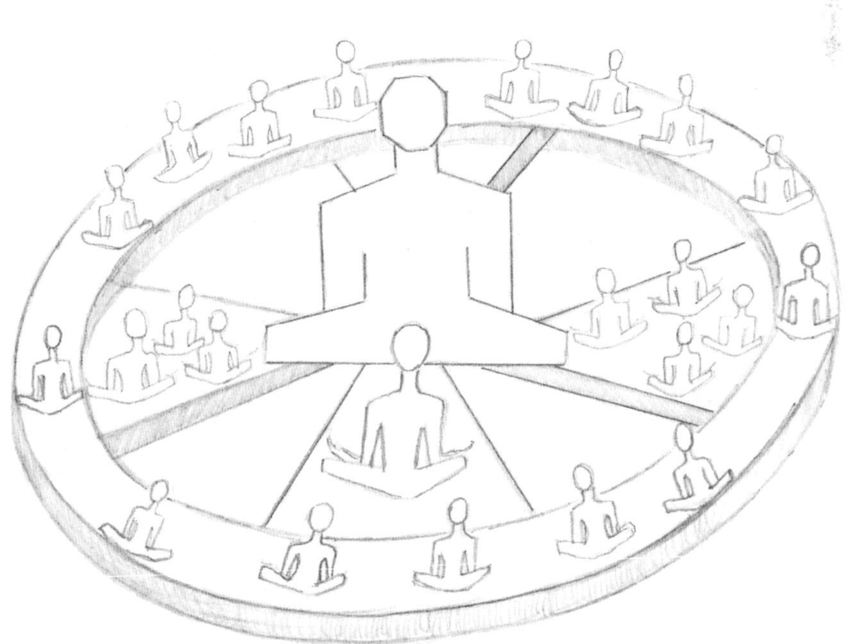

16 December 1998

During meditation, I get an insight into how the Creative Principle works.

At conception, birth of consciousness happens into the dense dimension, and at death, birth of consciousness happens into the subtle dimension.

What I understand of all that has gone by is:

The process of creation that I would have followed would be: When the One Source Consciousness starts to vibrate, pulsate, and move into a rhythm of self love of attraction and repulsion, contraction and expansion, fragmentation will take place. I as a fragmented, contracted, constricted and dense part of the One Source Consciousness would simultaneously move into the denser dimension of individualised union and drop into the dense womb. Thus, awareness contracts into consciousness, consciousness into energy, and energy into matter, creating an illusion that I am other than the Source.

At death, I drop back as the subtle dimensional consciousness into the cosmic womb and at birth I would drop back as dense dimensional consciousness into the individualised womb; so on, and on, from one womb into another! From subtle into the dense and from dense into the subtle.

With death, I would experience expansion and multi-dimensional awareness, and recognition of myself as the One Source Consciousness. With birth, I would experience contraction and fragmentation and enter an illusory state of existence. At death I would move out as consciousness, at birth I would get embodied and reach my dense state.

The whole exercise is gone through because as 'One Source Consciousness', Source does not know Itself. In order to fully know Itself as 'all of it', It must first experience Itself as not 'all of it', and in order to do that It has to create the other in relation to Itself. From the positive non-dual state of 'being', It enters into the negative dual state of 'becoming'. It enters into the field of the negative and positive polarities; of good and bad, right and wrong, conscious and unconscious etc.

19 December 1998

While we were sitting for evening meditation at the *Shibir* (retreat), I move as consciousness towards the *Guru* and I reach him; I see a window instead of the *Guru* and move out through him onto the hills of Mahabaleshwar. I come back with the sound of the *'Om'*.

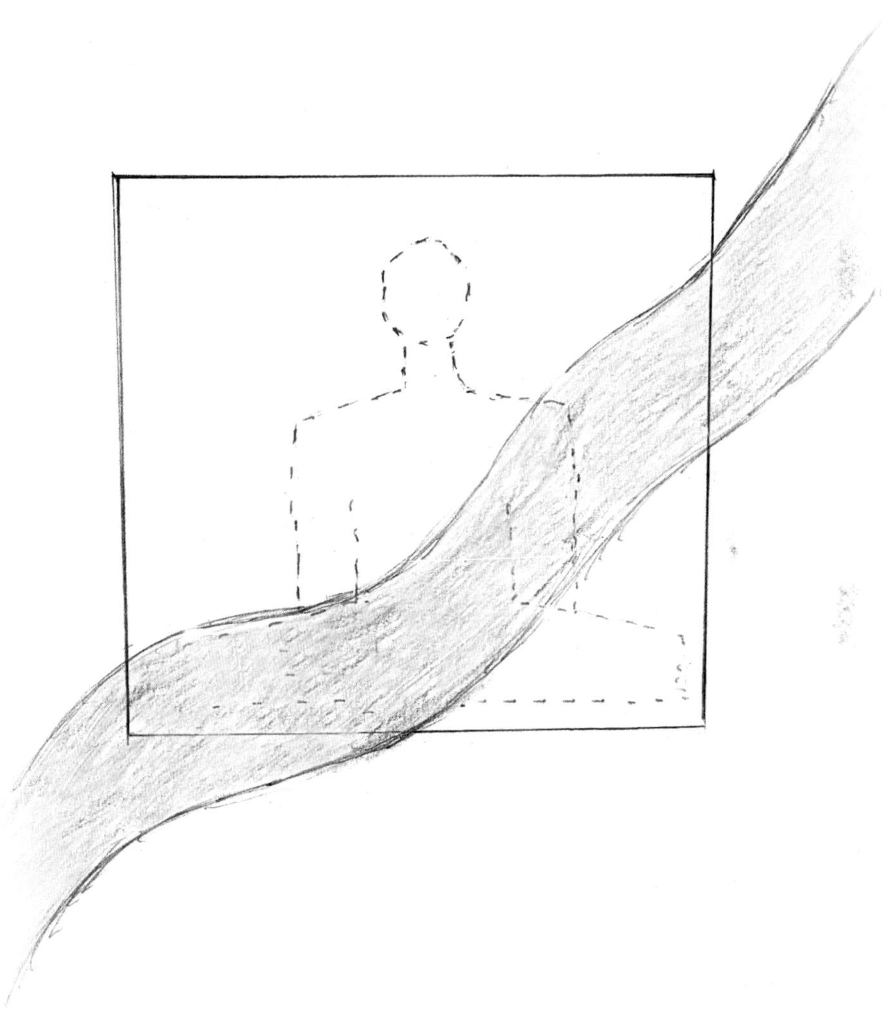

19 December 1998

A ball of shining thorns comes rotating towards my forehead. This then turns into a vibratory level of tiny waves. My *Ajna chakra* and *Manipur chakra* are rotating simultaneously with the in-between *chakras* missing, making me aware that I now operate at conscious level only. I see an open book now and then – a seal of light starts the movement of stamping the book.

I wonder whether it is the book of the *Hall of the Akashik Records* that is signed and sealed chapter by chapter.

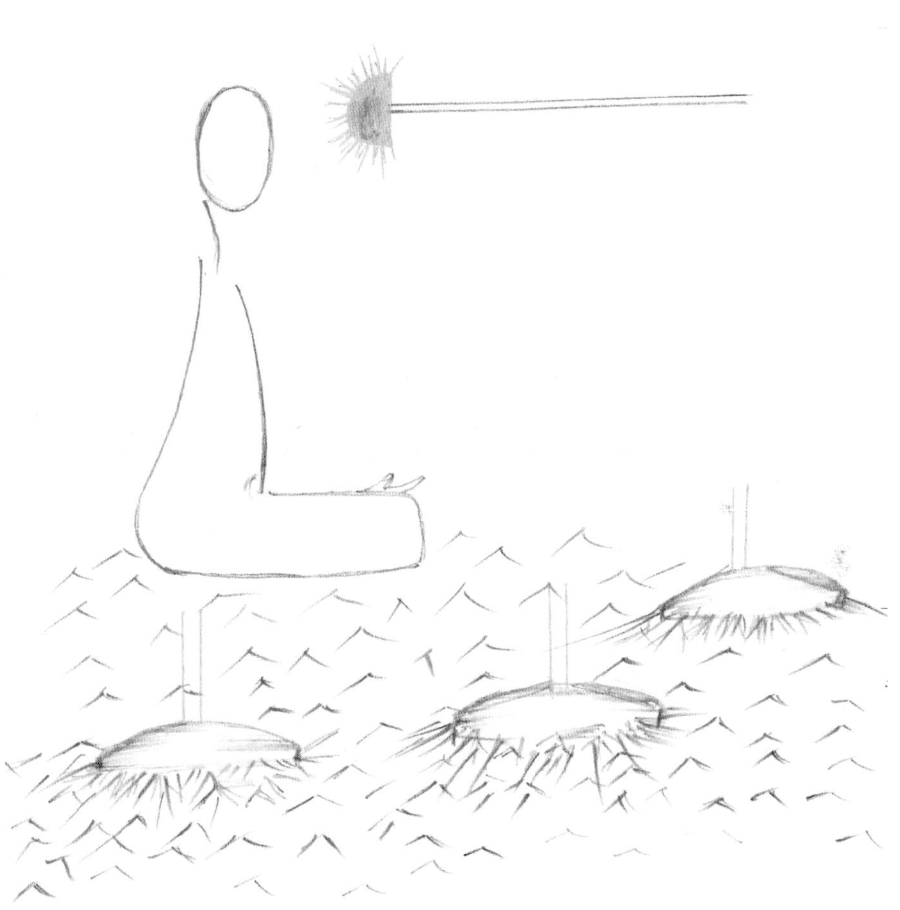

21 December 1998

Evening meditation: From the *Guru's Ajna chakra,* a tube extends to my *Ajna chakra.* I see a liquid of peacock colours flow from me towards the *Guru.* The right side of my head is reflecting splinters of light. The splinters start spreading in all directions. The splintered 'I' starts moving into a spherical shape along with the sound of *Guruji's Om,* following the process of dissolution and involution.

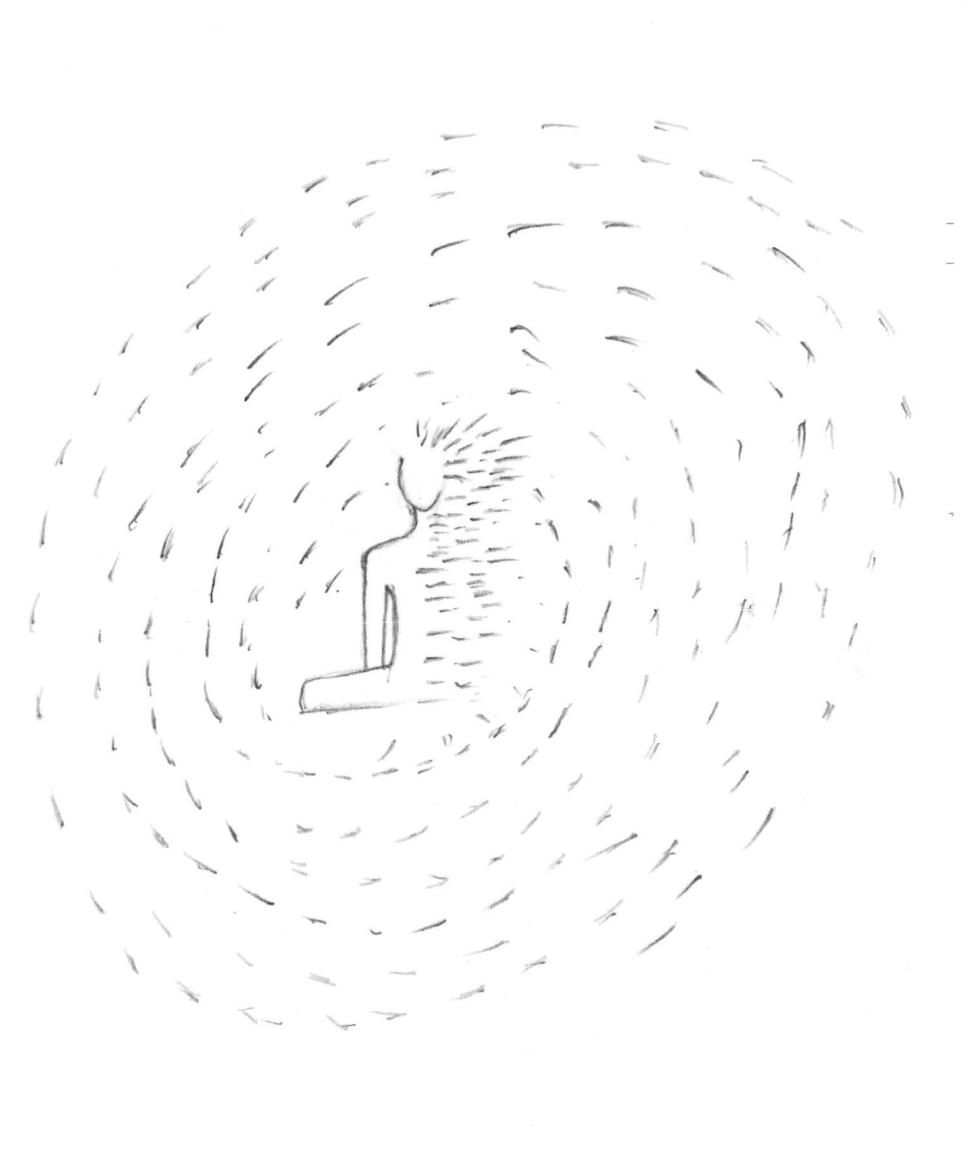

22 December 1998

Morning: On the left and the right side of the body, energy starts twirling around the *Sushumna nadi*. It is rising and moving in an upward direction. Both energies reach the head and move out. The vibrations give the impression of wings.

> R. A.: Santosh has here drawn a caduceus, the staff of Hermes with its double-twined snakes and the wings for a crown! It is the universal symbol for healing, and the prototype of all magical wands. Perhaps a symbol that Hermes could control these *Kundalini* energies consciously and use them to heal as well as to do magic with.

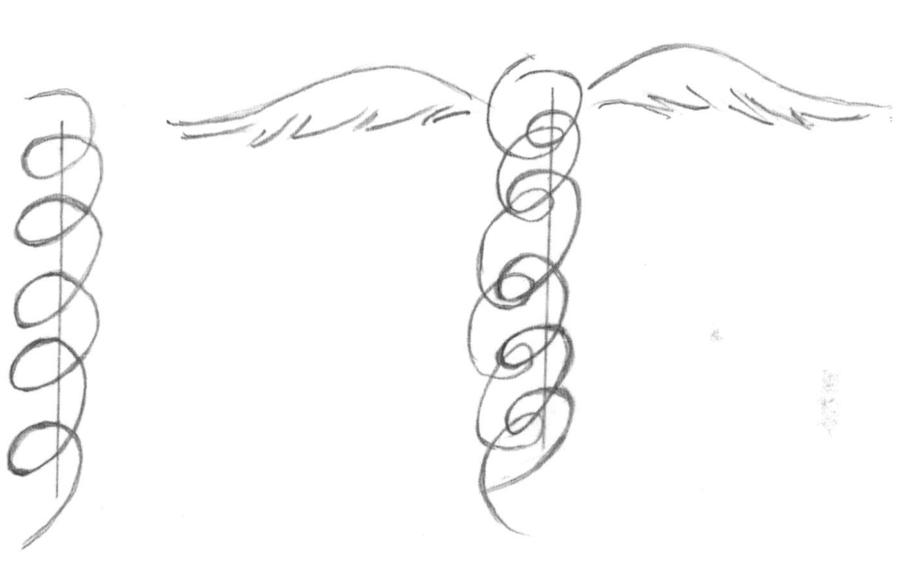

22 December 1998

Evening: During the evening meditation, I see the *Ida* and *Pingala* extending out of the body at an angle (Fig. 1). There are circles of energy twirling round them. The *Ida* and *Pingala* move towards each other (Fig. 2) and merge, forming *Sushumna,* the central channel (Fig. 3). Once the subtle channels are in place, I see consciousness start moving out of the *Guru's Ajna chakra,* sweeping over everyone sitting for meditation, and taking the Collective Consciousness along with it to the sound of *'Om'*.

This brings the powerful realisation that if one is able to connect with the *Guru* Consciousness, the work of the *Guru*/Master is made less strenuous.

The merging of the two channels would probably indicate a state of balance required for conscious existence. This balance is a natural happening when the consciousness rises, but once it comes into manifestation it gets into denser dimensions... from truth to illusion. Then, to get back into its natural state of balance, it has to work through several layers of dense mental data collected over lifetimes. It starts working towards recreating the balance it had lost. This it does through leading a life of discrimination and meditation and, in due course, reaching a level of complete detachment from all levels of mental dimensions and moving towards recognising itself as One Source Consciousness.

Once this is achieved, the consciousness is at rest and becomes the detached observer or Witness Consciousness and life is viewed as a series of events leaving just subtle surface impressions. As the detachment from the physical, mental, and emotional dimensions happens, there is stillness which in other words would mean, one gets into a state of *Samadhi* when Individual Consciousness is one with the Source Consciousness, a state during which one accesses all knowledge from the Void.

"The force of desire to experience is channelised through ida nadi, and the force which leads to action is channelised through pingala nadi. The two nadis have to be brought together; it is not a matter of eradicating them or suppressing them. The force channelised through both these nadis has to be channelised through sushumna. Only then can their influences be nullified. In hatha yoga we approach the problem of desire, vasana, impression, samskara, karma, action and reaction, by uniting these two channels of chitta and prana shakti."

– Muktibodhananda, op. cit., p. 483.

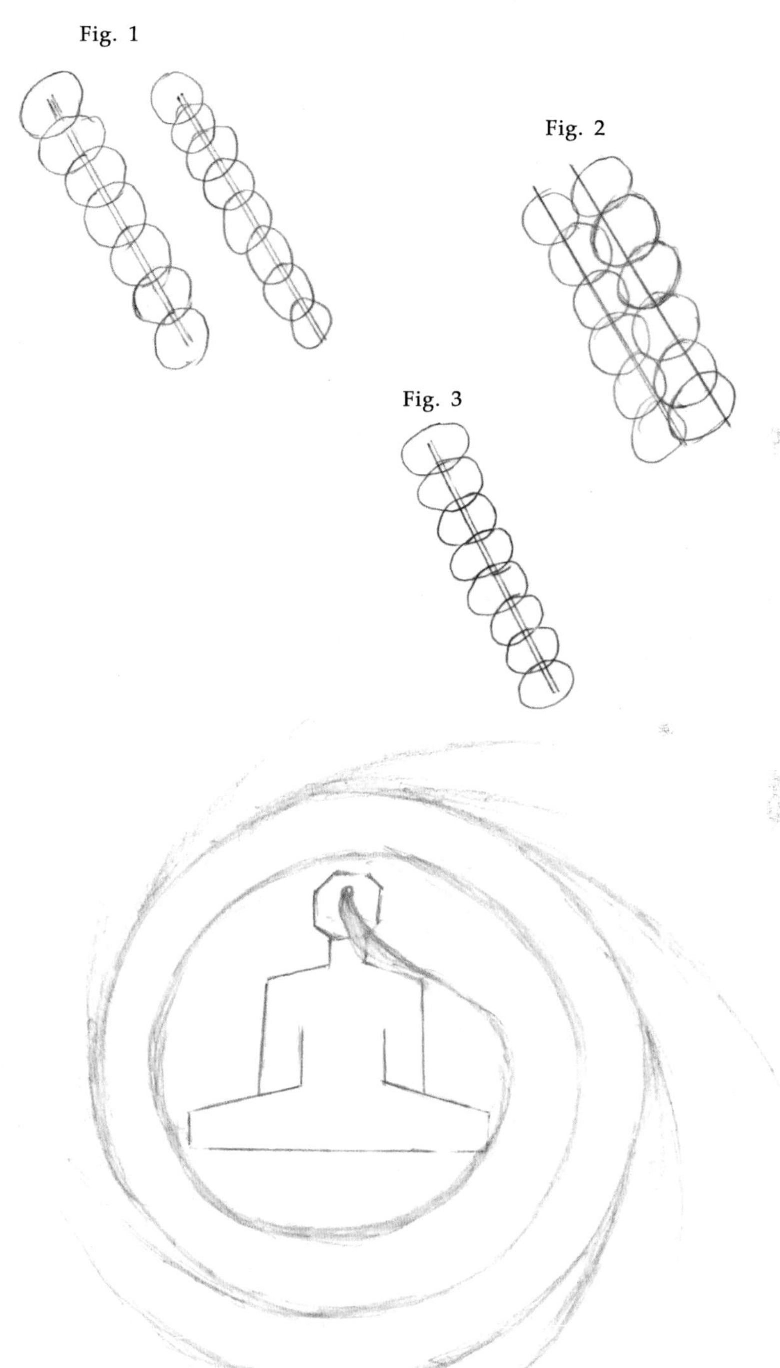
Fig. 1
Fig. 2
Fig. 3

7 January 1999

A *chakra* started moving in the right side of the head. A beam started from the left side of the head pointing behind, took a perpendicular path, pausing on either side of the head, doing a quick survey like a torch scanning, moving left and right. This activity is carried out at both the left and right temples. This activity led to a kind of disintegration and integration.

8 January 1999

I see a dark river flowing over my body (presumably blood). Ripples are being created by a rotary (instrument) of light moving over the black liquid, energising it. I can also see my ribcage and consciousness moving in as a yellow torch-head to settle in the right side.

Birth of a soul

What I seem to understand from the above visualisations is: Consciousness first demarcates the area or location of its manifestation. As fragmentation takes place, the subtle channels of *Ida* and *Pingala* manifest. The *Sushumna* gets active and ready for consciousness to move in. Blood in the form of an oily, dark liquid starts pouring in and it gets activated and energised with a beam of light. After the subtle channels and the *chakras* in the etheric body are in place, they attract the subtle matter of different elements. Since all creation is vibration, with deceleration, denseness starts to settle in. Consciousness then moves in through the *Sushumna* and places itself as a ball of light in the ribcage on the right side. This Individualised Consciousness, which is a part of the Source Consciousness residing within our body, is the one who fulfils all our hopes, wishes, and desires. It is our wish-fulfilling tree. "Ask and you shall receive." What is required of us is to live consciously otherwise we are creating a great deal of disharmony and dis-ease for ourselves.

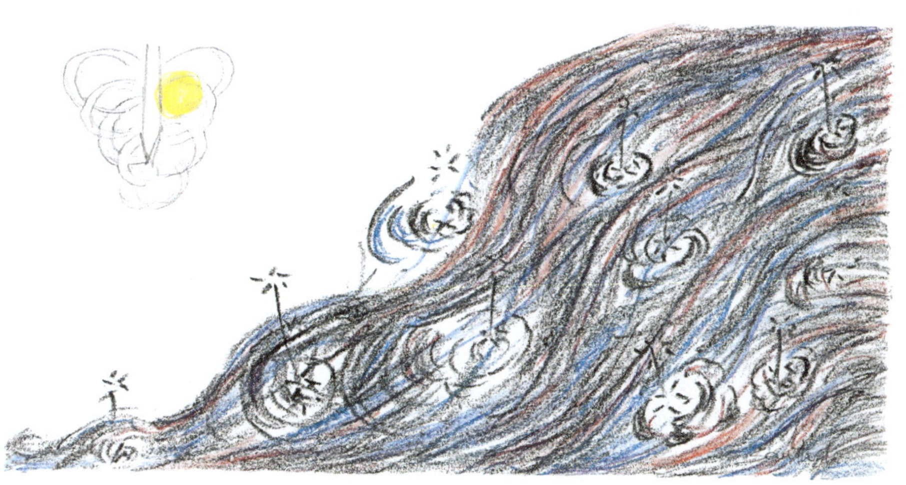

17 January 1999

During meditation, I suddenly become aware that my right brain and left brain are working simultaneously. My attention is more involved in the left brain, thinking of the book and how it will work. Then, my attention shifts to the right brain and I observe that it is working most efficiently, and to perfection. It is as if a record is playing, reciting all the affirmations in one part of the brain with the accompanying synchronisation of vibrations of the *chakra* in the other part. It is quite fascinating seeing both the right and left brain working simultaneously, without interfering with each other, in perfect rhythm. I (consciousness) could move from the right brain to the left brain without disturbance, planning, and looking at different options.

17 January 1999

I see a jug pouring milk into a bowl. Nothing strange in that, but I see the bowl in space facing downwards and the jug pouring milk into it from below. The placements are reversed. To me, it symbolises the flow of the *Kundalin*i energy moving from the *Muladhar chakra* to the *Sahasrar chakra*. I also seem to be assisted by an outside agency, and am made a recipient of more knowledge.

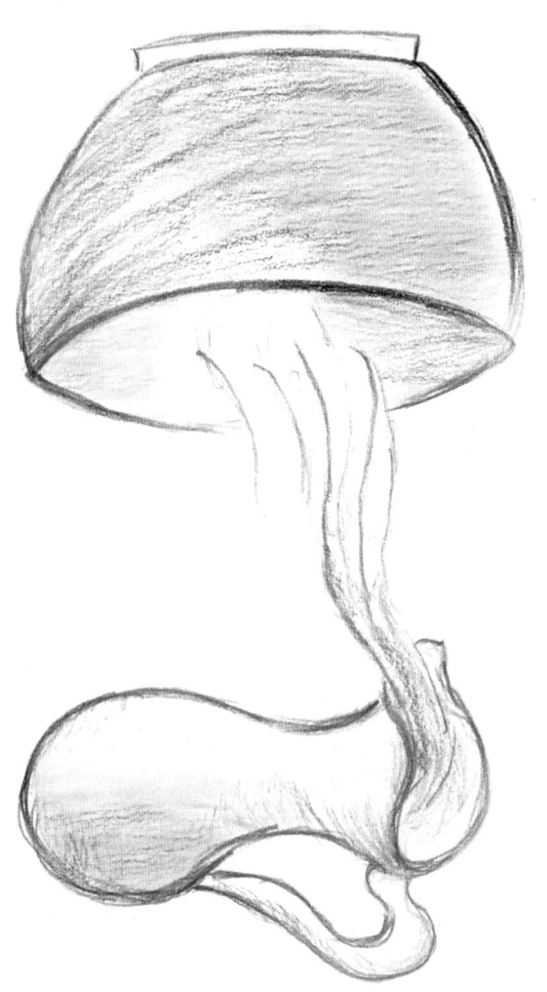

19 March 1999

I usually close my eyes when I do the exercises and the recitation of the affirmations. Today, I find after I open my eyes that I am facing the East instead of my usual South. This is a bit strange for me as nothing like this has happened before.

There is construction work going on in our vicinity. While meditating, consciousness identifies with the mud and rubble at the site.

20 March 1999

Today, I decide to do my exercises and affirmations facing the East. I am quite comfortable, though it feels a little strange.

I am having a nap in the afternoon. I have a dream. Two children and I are standing in front of a *pandit*. Turn by turn, we bend forward so that he can put a *tika* on our forehead. When I bend forward, he draws a *yantra* on my forehead. What does it signify?

> R. A.: This symbol has been used in many cultures to represent the labyrinth, in itself symbolic of the non-rational sections of the mind. It is one of the greatest archetypes known to humanity. The twists and turns of the labyrinth are an inevitable part of spiritual life. It does not matter how advanced you are spiritually; a new labyrinth springs up if you are not constantly vigilant. Also, the labyrinth is, according to western mystics, a physical device to activate the *chakras*. Moving in sequence through the levels of the maze automatically activate specific *chakras* as well as attune you to different levels of consciousness. The trick lies in being aware of such activation and utilising the energy released when one comes out of the maze. When the great mystery religions of Europe died out so did this arcane knowledge. It has been revived on a very small scale recently by Neo-pagans, but to reveal more here is not appropriate. The labyrinth is not, in a spiritual sense, a space where you get hopelessly lost and confused. Quite the contrary, in fact. You enter the maze, which is a physical symbol of being spiritually lost and emotionally confused, and find your Self. There is a difference, a great one, in this inversion. It is a field of *sadhana* and a potent symbol for life itself.

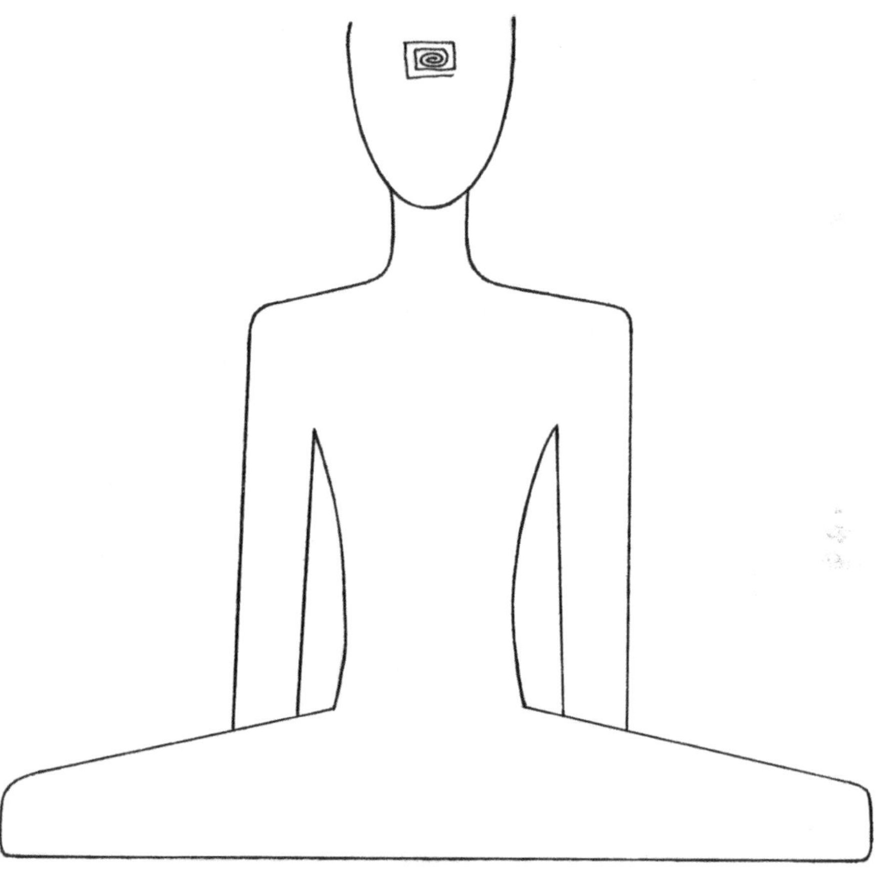

22 March 1999

4:30 am: The body just feels vibration, there is a gentle tingling all over. There is pressure at a certain point, midway in the right arm.

7:30 am: I do the exercises facing south-east. During meditation, I feel the body undergoing a certain vibratory change. What I think is happening is: it is not that the body moves to another vibratory plane, but its own vibration changes to move to another level of existence.

6 April 1999

Group meditation: I feel in the left brain above the temple, as if a pointed instrument is pushing at the brain tissue until it stretches. There is pain. I relax and allow the procedure to complete itself. This somehow reminds me of the unicorn.

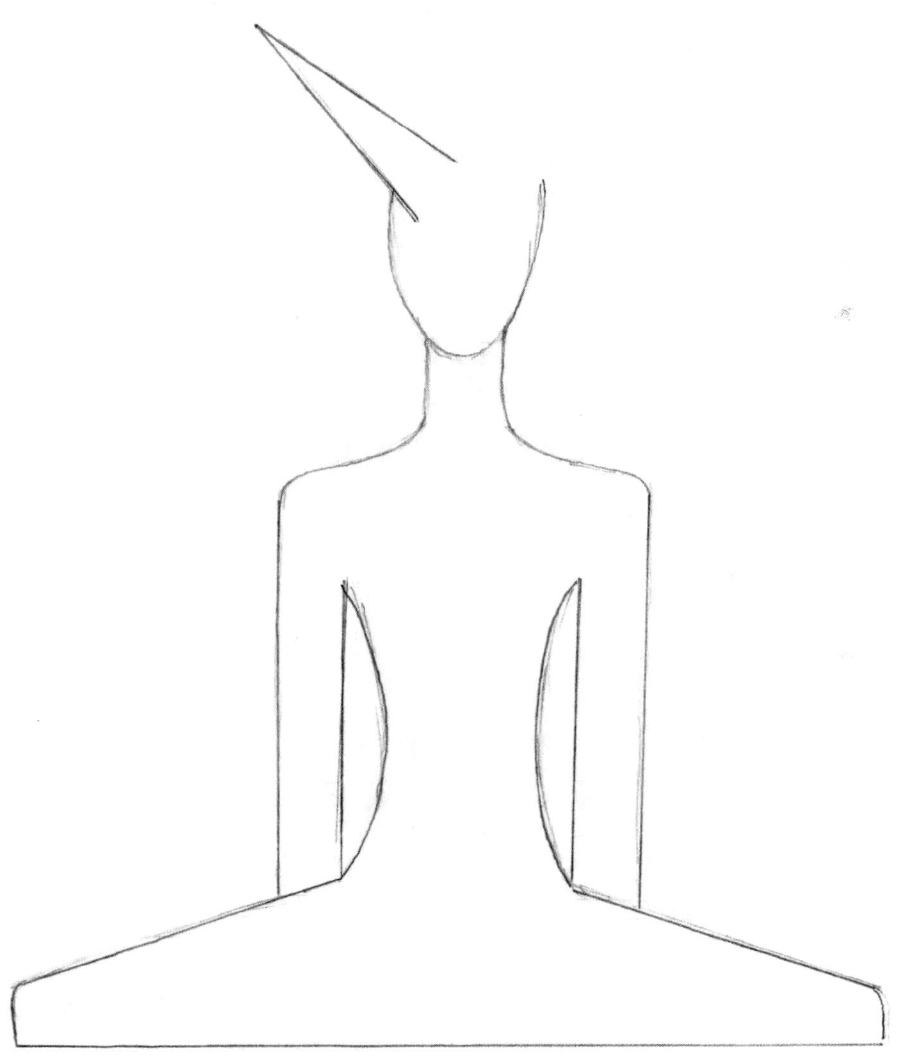

7 April 1999

I feel painful pressure on top of the head towards the right. I stay with it.

2 May 1999

Instead of Tuesday, we had the group meditation today i.e. Sunday. I experienced a total feeling of lightness; all the denseness seemed to have disappeared. Instead of the nose, it felt as if I had a small tube through which the breath was moving. The whole body was a beautiful, green plant that would open and close to the rhythm of the *chakras.* I see the *Guru* as a gray-coloured mound; there are green-coloured creepers climbing over him till he is covered with them.

> R. A.: This is a common theme in the mythology of the Hindus, the *Guru* or meditator who is so absorbed in his *sadhana* that he gets covered with a mound of earth upon which greenery begins to flourish. The creepers stand for all those aspirants who will be nourished by the *Guru's* wisdom but they will rarely know his full nature, which has to remain concealed for their own sake. It also indicates a total merging into the natural realm, by which the *Guru* is indistinguishable from Nature – always one of the finest *Gurus.*
>
> This strongly brings home the necessity of a *Guru* if one wants to be a serious aspirant on the path of spiritualism.

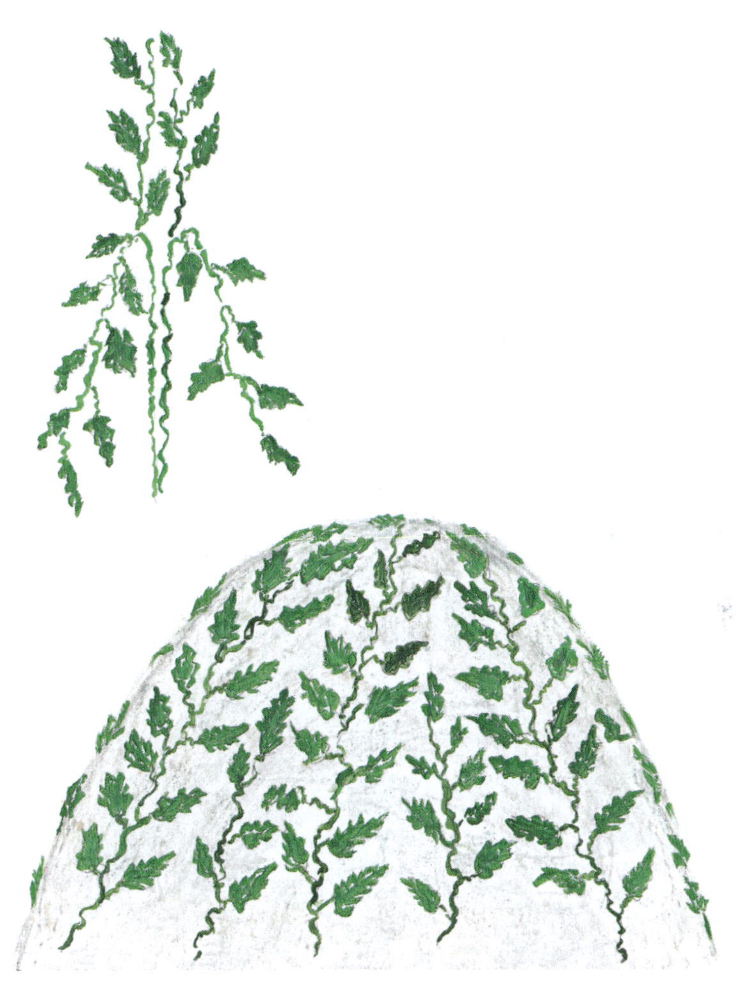

10 May 1999

I get into some sort of a spaceship with *Guruji*. I am moving anti-clockwise as consciousness, much above a blanket of stars which move clockwise.

9 July 1999

During the exercise, when I bend my neck forward with the chin down, there is a dull *nada* sound, whereas, while bending from waist forward and backwards the sound takes on a higher pitch.

When I sit for meditation, my chest and back are checked with a stethoscope.

Does it mean a new phase is about to start?

23 July 1999

There is a change in the body vibrations. These vibrations are in the body, more like a gentle current passing through. The feeling is as if the body is made of tiny balls.

1 October 1999

I see that my body is a pole of light with flourescent colours of energy rotating at the two ends. I suppose this is the way I would look without the covering of my dense physical, mental, and emotional data.

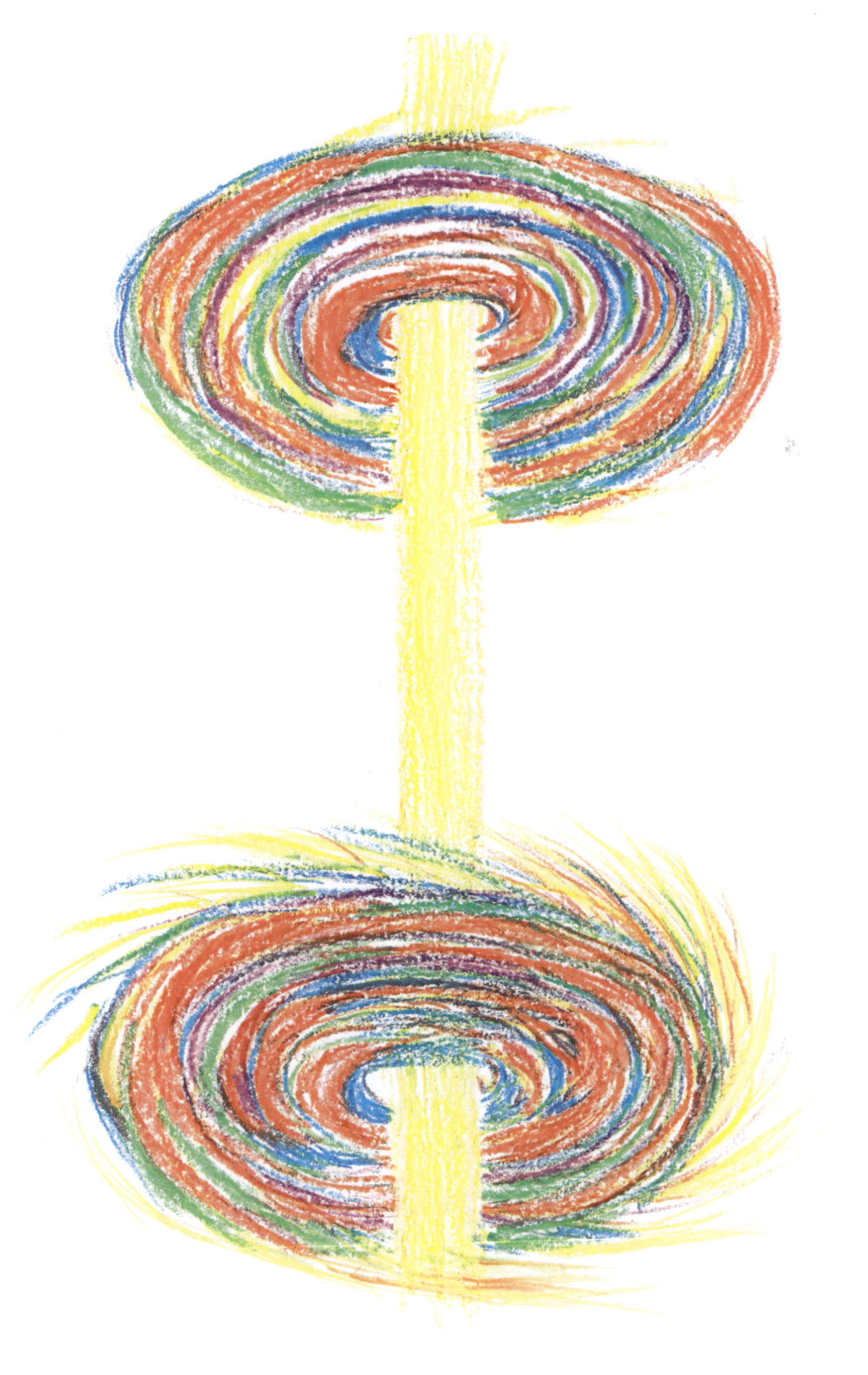

4 October 1999

During meditation, my head opens up and starts to disperse as balls of energy. Are my atoms being rearranged?

11 October 1999

A peculiar phase has started; my hearing is affected. There is no sound in the subtle ear. There is complete silence within and without.

I am completely focused in the *Ajna chakra.*

13 October 1999

The stillness continues. Consciousness alternates between the *Ajna,* Heart and *Manipur chakra.*

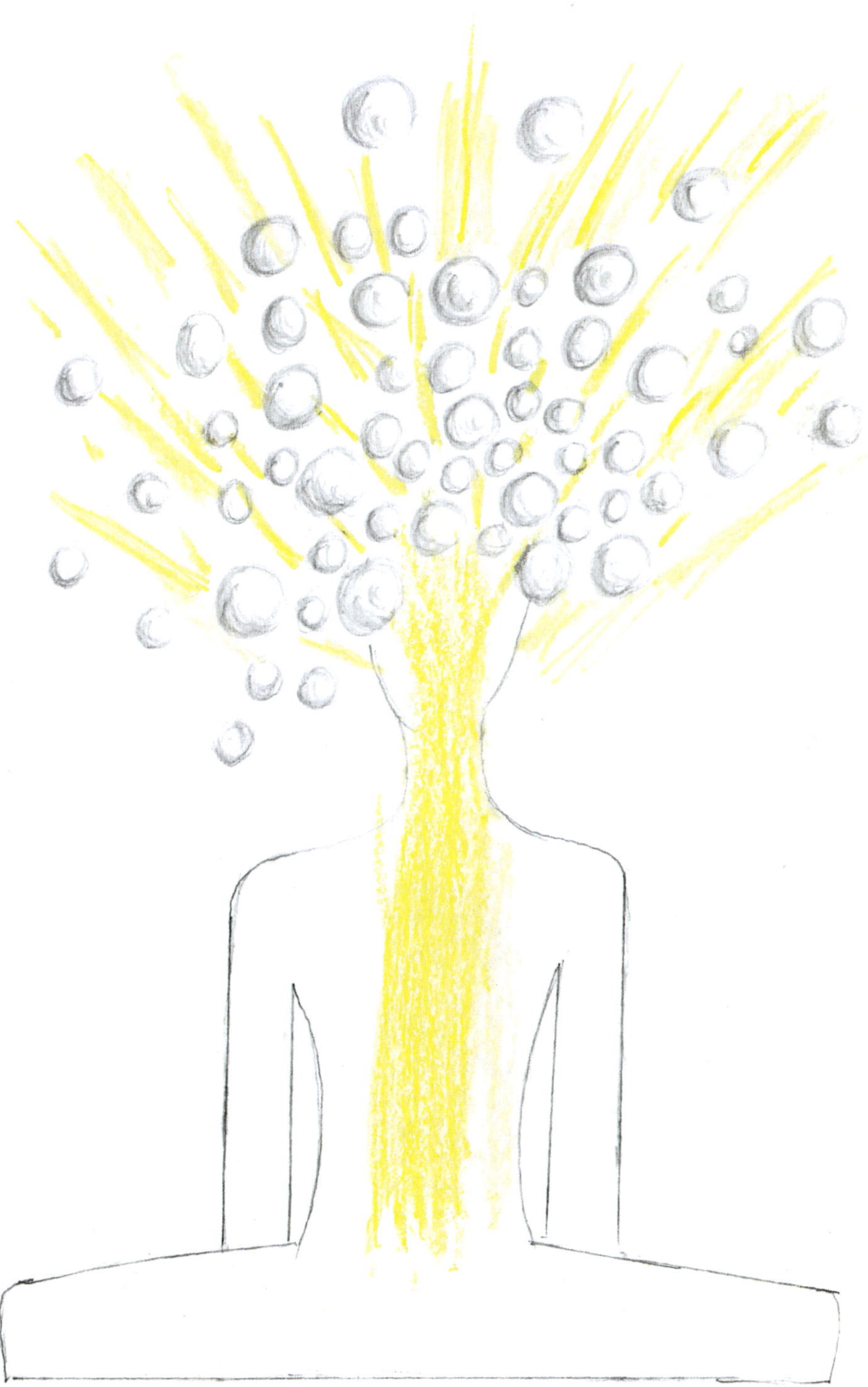

14 October 1999

The focus at the *Ajna chakra* was fixed and shining. It was throwing a beam of light. The *Manipur* is active and starts expanding till I am only light.

When these two *chakras* are functioning in harmony and synchronicity, the aspirant would then lead a balanced life. In other words, the *Ganpati* principle would be dominant in her/his life. Meaning, she/he would not be bogged down by life's pleasures and pains, and would view every stressful or happy situation as a play of consciousness.

15 October 1999

The fixed state continues, interspersed with meaningless conversations with individuals, known and unknown.

Do I fall asleep and wake up? I am also aware of looking into a blank, lighted forehead as if it is a screen. Sometimes I am fixed in the chest.

22 October 1999

Today, I am consciously attentive to some letters being pointed out to me. I nod my head to indicate that I understand. The script is unfamiliar and written downwards like Chinese. The figures are more like numbers.

My left forearm moves out and the palm of the hand faces me. It is dotted with red and blue.

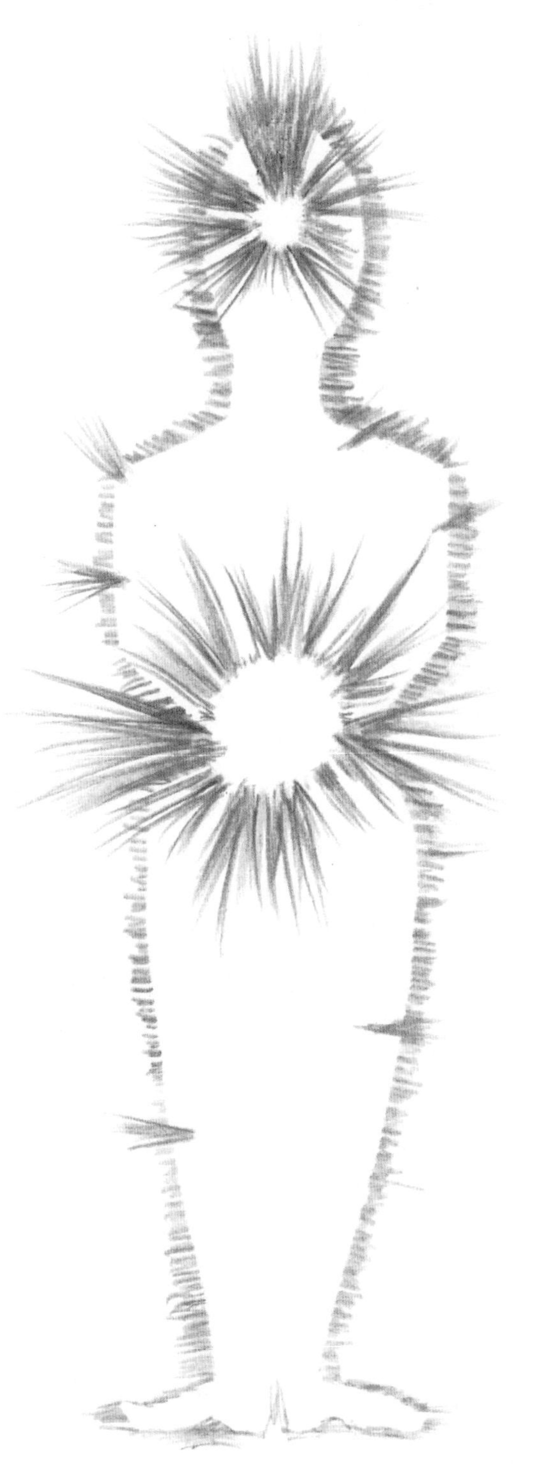

30 November 1999

Group meditation: Guruji verbally guided our consciousness to a certain level.

My *Ajna chakra* focused at the *Guru's Muladhar,* tracing the course of energy to his *Sahasrar chakra,* coming back into my Crown *chakra.* I become a straight rod of energy, and I am the wind and the autumn leaves.

The other aspirants experienced a feeling of bliss and a vision of me dressed in red.

17 December 1999

4:30 am: I see the Source (cosmos) form two hands that move in the slow motion of clapping. Then it starts to dance as if in celebration. I wonder as to what is there to celebrate! Then I see *Guruji* in a white van – wearing a cream-coloured *kurta.* He is greeting everyone with joint hands as the car moves along.

16 February 2000

I do not focus too much on the completion of the affirmations now, because it delays the process of my getting into deep meditation. I move in and out of awareness. Occasionally, thoughts flit by.

22 February 2000

There are gold ornaments lying on the floor. Someone picks all up and consciously leaves a small gold bead behind. A bird comes, fluttering and hopping, and picks it up in its beak. The fluttering and hopping of the bird is created in my right temple.

A spoon is put in my mouth with something in it; I don't know whether it is my hand holding the spoon or some other. From my chest, a small bird flutters out.

23 February 2000

Consciousness identifies with a shootout somewhere.

Someone shoots me in the right side of my forehead; I crumble. I feel a rope-like movement of energy in my back, moving from the base upwards.

23 February 2000

There is a meeting of descending and ascending energy. There is no feeling of a body from the chest upwards. There is no neck and head. Instead, the entire area of the abdomen and above is only light, and what is visible is a good-sized pendulum moving like a temple bell beyond the *Sahasrar chakra* (Crown *chakra*). Fascinating! The Individualised Consciousness remains as a shining flame ready to merge with the consciousness at rest or the Source.

Going through the above experience, and contemplating and meditating on it, has cleared the process of my thought completely. I recall *Guruji's* words each time I would ask him to explain the meaning of my experience. His response would be: "Wait, it will unfold in time."

I realise that once the dense body starts to become subtle, once the denseness starts to fall off, what remains is a drop, the Individual Consciousness, which is ready to fall into the ocean of Source Consciousness. Till such time as that happens, it will continue to be a pendulum and toll as a resounding bell either from a church steeple or a temple, and be the wake-up call for those ready to know themselves and move on to the road of self-discovery, thus getting out of the cycle of birth and death, from subtle consciousness to dense consciousness and from dense consciousness to subtle and so on.

I marvel every time I get an insight into the astuteness of our *rishis*. They created a symbol for everything they experienced at the subtle level. The human body is given the symbol of a temple and a church; with the bell symbolising the Source residing within us. Just as we go into a temple and we see and worship the deity, if we were to go within ourselves, we would come face to face with that part of the Source that is residing within us as Individual Consciousness.

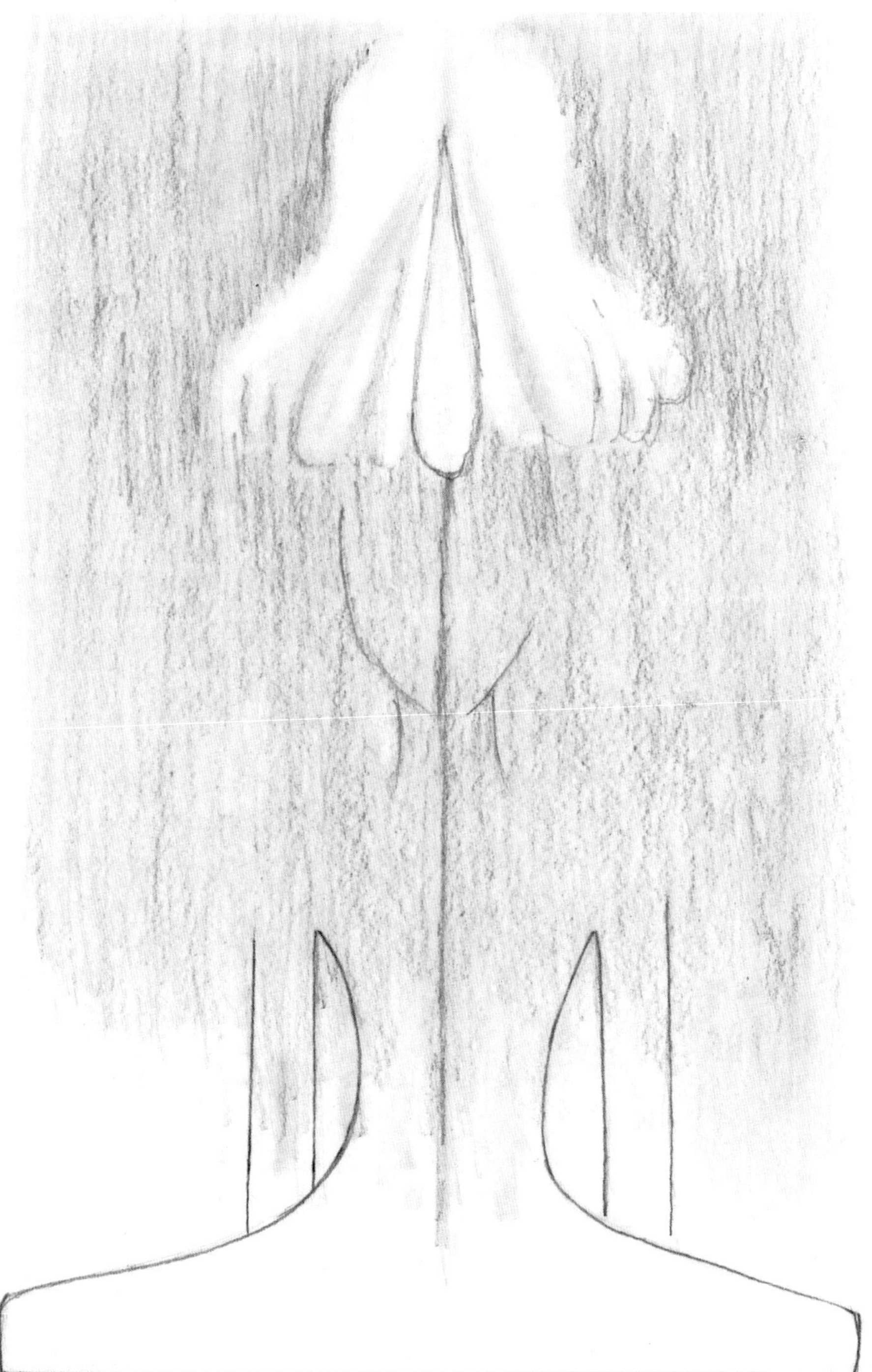

23 February 2000

The centre point of the *trishul,* the symbol of the *Shaivites,* also represents Consciousness, with the rod symbolising the shining *Sushumna.* The *trishul* is always carried by them or placed next to wherever they are sitting; it automatically raises the consciousness to the Crown *chakra* and above.

I give below, a few lines from the affirmation that goes with my experience of the visual:

"My Body – the temple, the temple of the Living God, the temple of the God that lives within me – that is alive within me. I stand in reverence before the wisdom pent up in the very substance of my body – and I pledge myself, I vow, that from this moment henceforth nothing that I shall do, or say, or think, shall injure or abuse this temple of the Living God, my body."

The book of my unfoldment makes me wonder at the process of my experience. I am sure the knowledge that is channeled through me has a purpose. I offer my humble thanks and gratitude to my *Guru,* to the Masters, and the Higher Forces for finding this body-mind intellect worthy of their purpose.

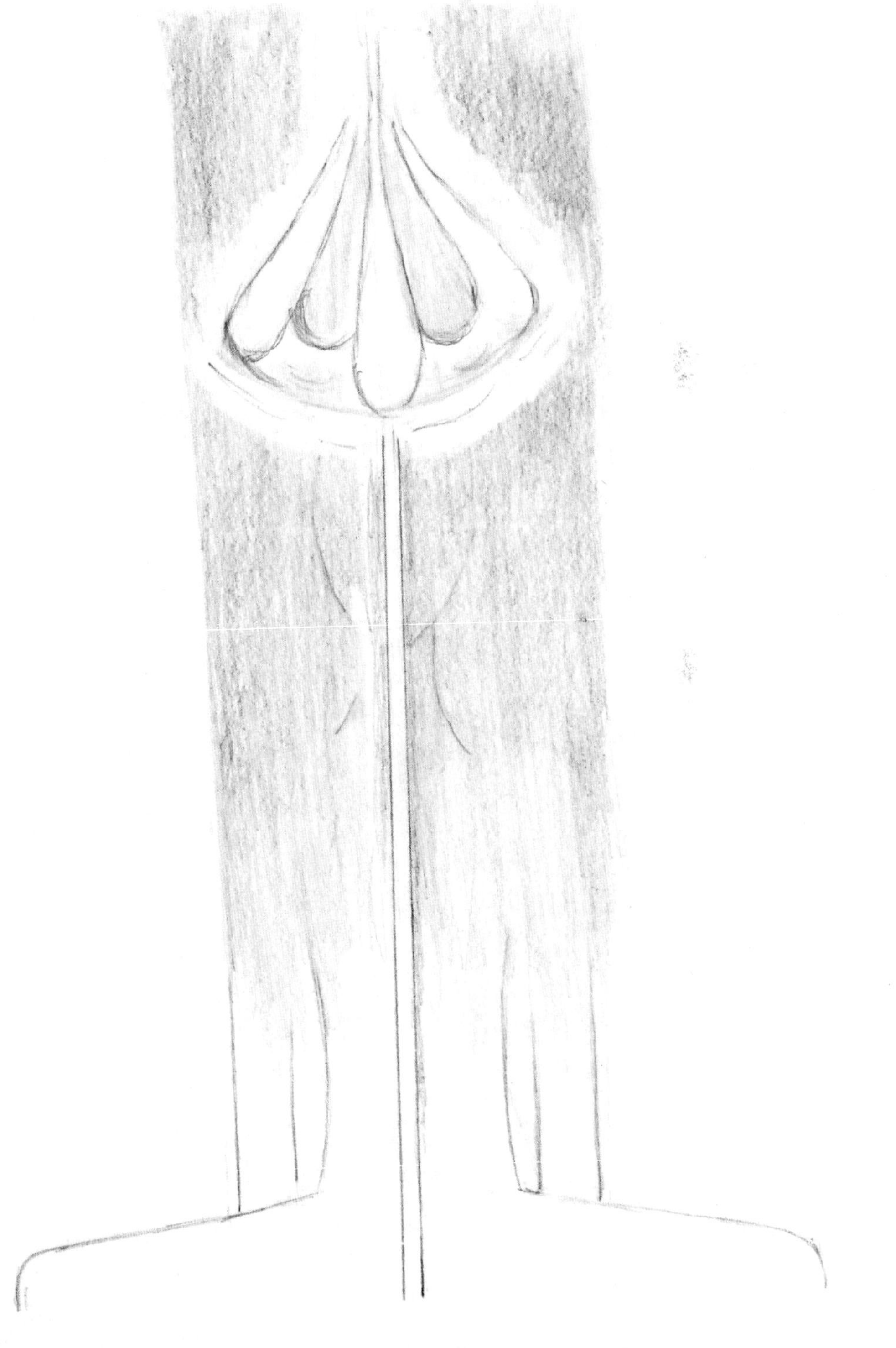

24 February 2000

Death & After

The Ultimate/Final Expansion; process of merging before the stillness.

Sitting down for meditation in the early hours of the morning, I get the experience of what would happen at the death of the physical body, or the ultimate expansion:

A beam of light extends from the *Ajna chakra,* traces a path up the forehead for consciousness to move out from the centre at the top of the head and pierce the cosmos, creating a ripple and merging with the Source Consciousness. Simultaneously, all the *chakras* in the different parts of the body start unwinding, expanding, and merging with the different elements they are composed of. What is left moving is a subtle form resembling the *yin yang* symbol at the *Manipur chakra* level. It is probably a bundle of unresolved desires waiting to attach itself when the subtle consciousness once again moves towards the denser dimension of existence.

"The image of integration is the unio mystica, the fusion of opposites. This is a time of communication between the previously experienced dualities of life. Rather than night opposing day, dark suppressing light, they work together to create a unified whole, turning endlessly one into the other, each containing in its deepest core the seed of the opposite."

– 'Osho Zen Tarot – The Transcendental Game of Zen'. St. Martin's Press, 175 Fifth Avenue, New York, 1994. Second Edition, p. 30.

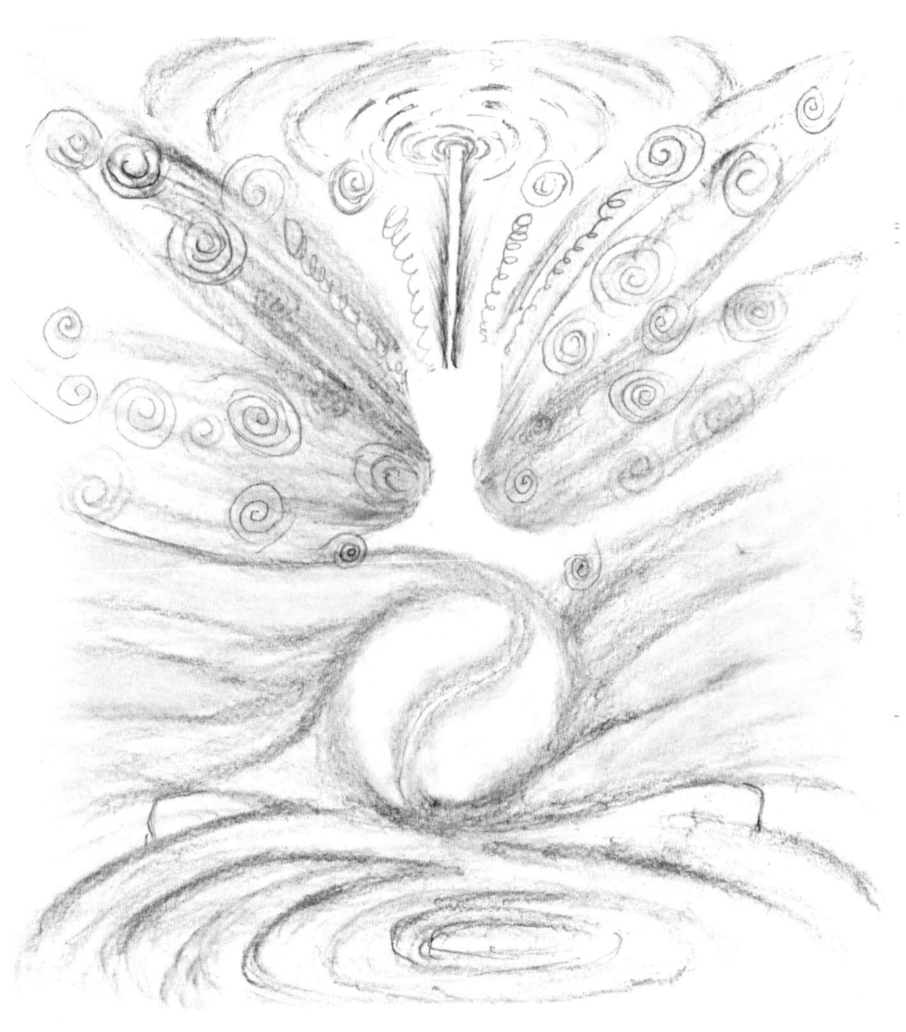

23 April 2000

After the final expansion and merging, I now invariably experience myself standing on a pedestal. However, on physical verification, I see that I am very much on the floor.

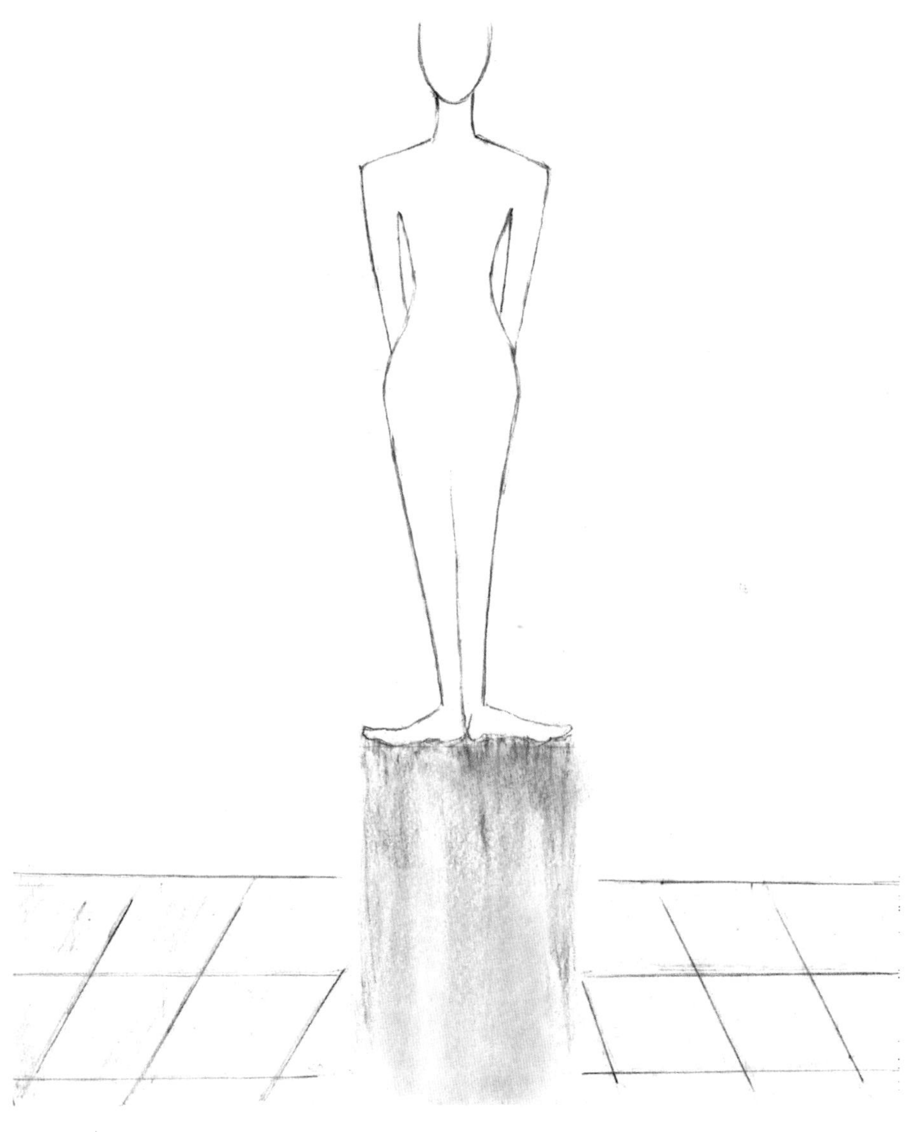

23 April 2000

During meditation, I move as a sheet of consciousness. When I reach a certain level, I am showered first with white light and then with rainbow colours, and merge with the consciousness as a whole.

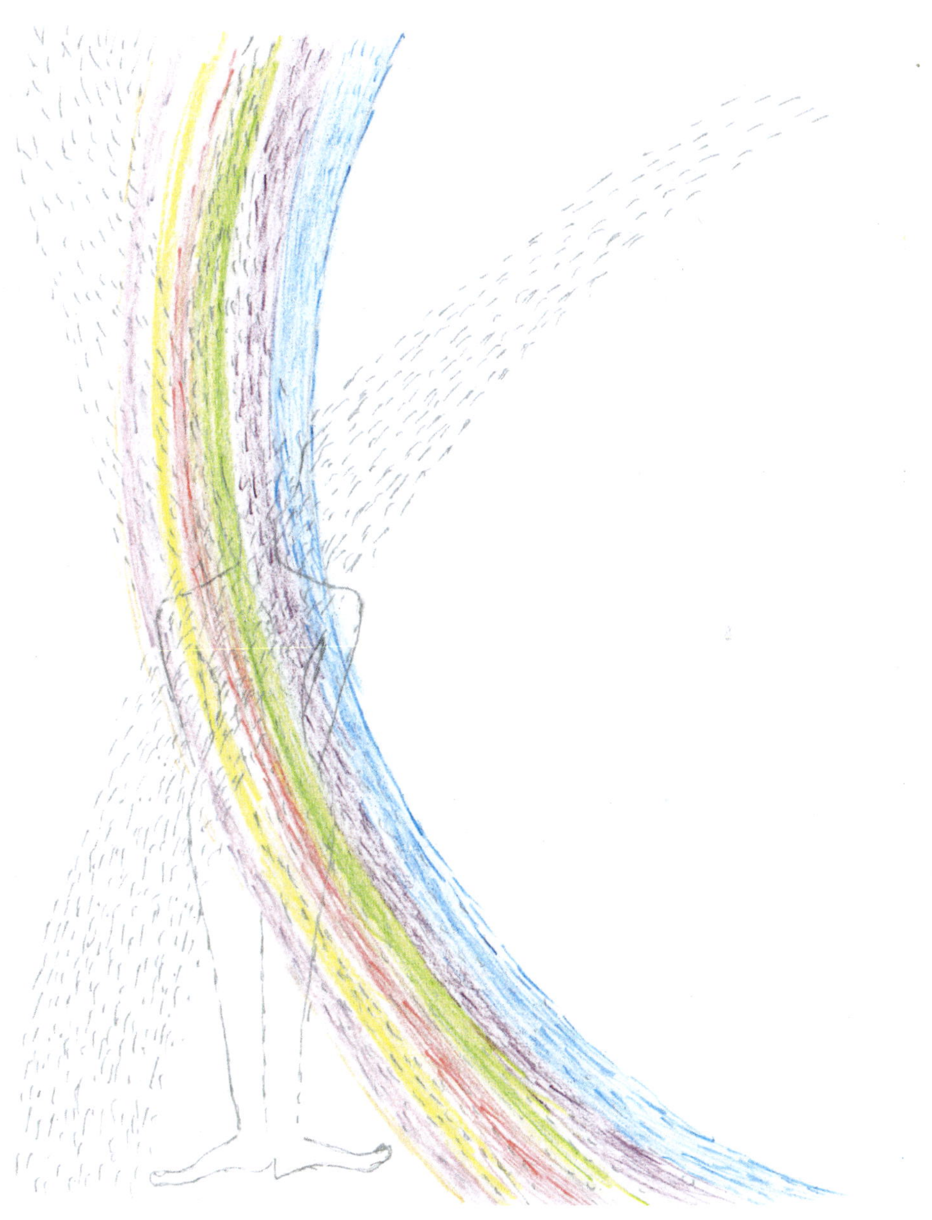

25 April 2000

During meditation, I see in the deep blue void the form of the *Guru*. The form is bathed in light, the head is also throwing rays of light. Slowly and steadily, the form starts sinking into the void and then disappears. I assumed that the journey of unfoldment, which had started for me on 1st November, 1995 with the manifestation of the *Guru,* was now complete and the *Guru* principle deemed it appropriate to leave me on my own to move on at my own pace.

This knowledge, this experience, and this creativity is possible when the Guru-Disciple relationship manifests at the deepest level of existence and transcends duality, and one can remain receptive to the impulses flowing from the Divine from within and without.

Would the Source reveal itself so completely to an individual? Why? Is it in preparation for the times that are to come? Are we moving towards a time where we will have to have a different understanding? Does it mean that henceforth, our evolution will start with the awareness of Source Consciousness? Will I get an answer to my questions? Yes.

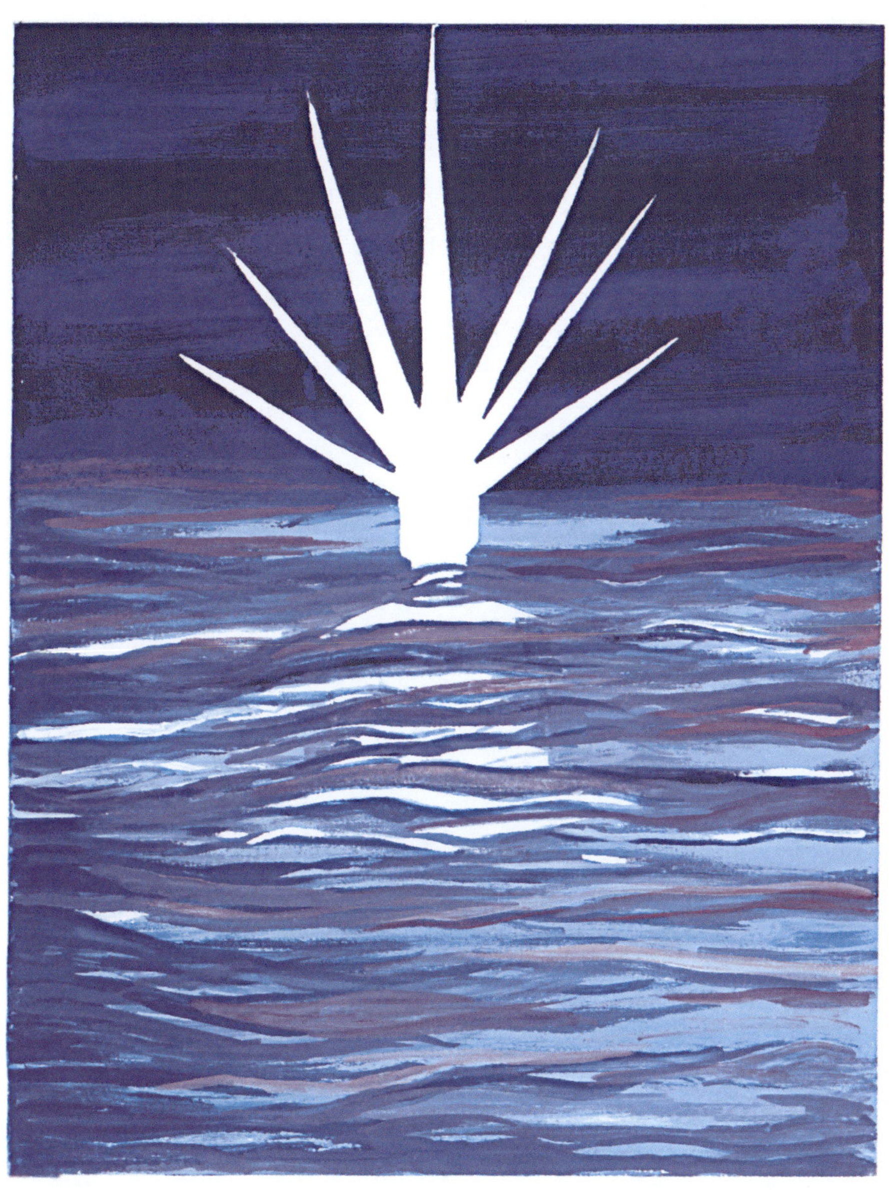

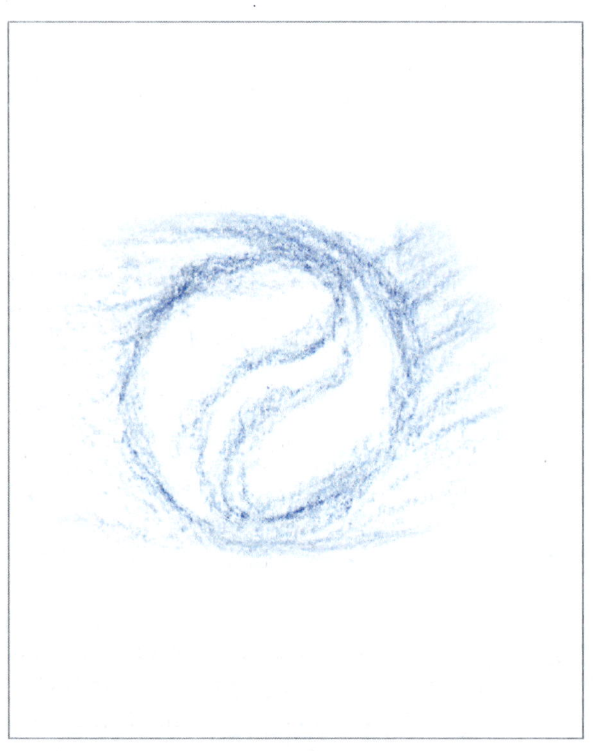

SOUL-MATE

What is a soul-mate?

"A beam of light extends from the *Ajna chakra,* traces a path up the forehead for consciousness to move out of the centre at the top of the head and pierce the cosmos, creating a ripple and merging with the Source Consciousness. Simultaneously, all the *chakras* in the different parts of the body start unwinding, expanding, and merging with totality or the different elements of what they are composed of. What is left moving in a *yin yang* fashion, at the *Manipur chakra* level, is probably a bundle of unresolved desires waiting to attach itself when the subtle consciousness once again moves towards the denser dimension of existence."

The fully integrated consciousness would, at death, merge with the Source Consciousness but, since embodiment involves limitation, the embodied consciousness, no matter how expanded, is bound to collect some baggage. This data collection can be through compassion, imbedded conditioning to cultural patterns, or one's own guilt or self-created value system. Even though there is no clinging attachment to this baggage of collected data of hopes and fears and unfulfilled desires and aspirations, it still must exhaust itself. And, for that, it must await its turn to attach itself to consciousness when it is in motion. It may so happen that only a part of the bundle of *karma* or desires manages to get onto the bandwagon and propel itself into embodiment, leaving a part of itself to await its turn in the movement of consciousness. According to our time-frame, it can happen even every thirty years, and at different levels of social structure. When the beings of the same baggage meet, a sense of completion arises and they recognise each other as soul-mates. The *karma* is being worked out at different levels, and if one moves towards it consciously, a time may come when there is no more baggage and complete dissipation of that particular bundle.

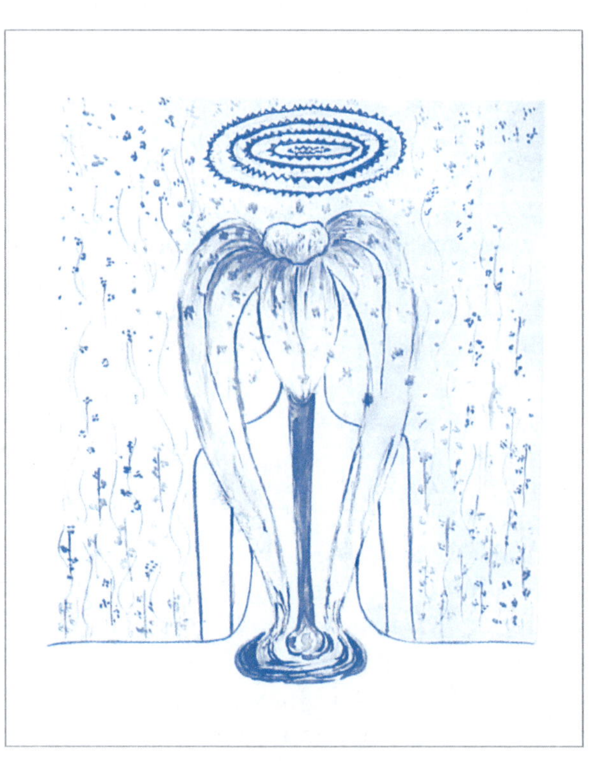

MEDITATION

You get different messages when the question arises as to what are you supposed to do when you sit down for meditation. Some say, "concentrate and focus," while others say, "drive out all thoughts," and still others say, "watch your breath." What do you do when you forget to watch your breath? This leads to stress and frustration for the raw aspirant, because he really does not understand the meaning of 'meditation'.

The purpose of meditation is to help a person become free of stress, and this can only happen if his body-mind and spirit are in harmony. Consciousness oscillates between the two hemispheres of the brain i.e. the right and left cortical regions. The left side is the logical mind and the right side is the creative mind. The left side of the brain can be termed as negative polarity and the right side as the positive polarity. The dense physical, emotional, and mental dimension is dominated by the left life-negative polarity that becomes more active during meditation, thus accelerating the process of shifting and throwing up thoughts that have been stored in the deep recesses of the brain. This also indicates that 'meditation' is working and fulfilling its purpose of gradually bringing the two polarities (the right and left brain) to a balance. *Guruji* says, "Do not struggle with the mind. Thinking is a vital part of the human condition and instead of fighting, resisting, and identifying with your thoughts, you should become the detached observer of whatever thinking is taking place."

By bringing awareness to the mind and allowing the thoughts to be as they are, not getting entangled with them or entering into a dialogue, the mind will become more balanced. This is not something that will happen overnight. A process has been set in motion with meditation, and it will take a great deal of practice and patience in order to see results. First, the three bodies of the dense physical, emotional, and mental dimensions will have to be brought into balance. Out of these, the mental dimension has the maximum layers of stored data that needs to be processed, and complete detachment from these layers will happen gradually.

Once you get into a programme, and a regular routine of practice and meditation is observed, the process of balancing begins. Initially, there is constant and automatic undirected thinking and throwing up of life-negative dualistic data of right and wrong, good and bad, happy and sad etc. embedded in the subconscious; there is no synchronicity or coordination in the two brain hemispheres. The left life-negative data of events and experiences overshadows the right life-positive data of awareness. At such times, we find ourselves stressed, distracted, unhappy, or fearful. Then there is directed thinking. This means that we direct the mind through empowering thoughts/affirmations of non-dualistic nature, and along with being in the energetic field of the *Guru,* a shift starts taking place and one moves towards balance between the two hemispheres.

Once this balance is achieved then the left and the right polarities begin to synchronise and life-positive polarity becomes dominant. The earlier confusion gives way to expanded awareness leading to a sense of calmness. As balance between the two polarities is maintained through focus, in due course, Witness Consciousness opens up. At this stage, what remains of the mind is surface impressions of irrelevant data as focus shifts between the negative and now dominant positive dimension, causing no stress or confusion. It is more like sitting by the sea-shore and watching the traffic go by. Once all data is processed without our involvement in it, what transpires is 'stillness'. This is the subtlest level of the mind where one is not becoming, but just being.

Guruji says that it is not important to have any experiences or states; what is important is to be ever watchful and vigilant so that whenever undirected thinking takes place we gently return back to the breath or whatever chosen means of focus. Being aware is the simplest way to success in meditation.

Chapter Seven

CONCLUSION

After nearly seven years of practicing *Brahma Vidya,* I realise that it is fortunate that when I joined the course, I had no idea of what I was getting into. To me, getting into a regular routine of exercise, and learning the affirmations by heart meant going back to school. Though I enjoyed going to school, I definitely did not enjoy the routine of study. The best possible way was to finish learning whatever I had to learn, in the shortest possible time. I tended to follow the same pattern with *Brahma Vidya,* and it is my good luck that the *Guru* sensed this and supported me by guiding me through a most thrilling adventure, where my curiosity was kept alive and charged to a level where I would be enthusiastically looking forward to new mountains to climb and devils to subdue, so that I could see what is on the other side.

The adventure was also the result of not being an absolute clear channel, for *Kundalini* is only felt if you do not have a very clear passage and it meets with resistance. This resulted in my getting to know *Kundalini* most intimately. If the passage was completely clear and *Kundalini* would have moved smoothly, I would not have experienced the various shifts and transendence from one level to another. My sensitivity and focus was raised to the optimum level so that I would be totally attentive in order to register and absorb its functioning in the human body-mind intellect.

Having moved very gently initially, giving me a visual knowledge of itself and its movement within my physical body, a time came when serious work was to be done. This was to be done in its own territory of the 'etheric body'. Unless the etheric centres were working properly, the related physical organs would also be malfunctioning. Since I had no knowledge to fathom what was taking place, my intuition took over and I became a keen observer of what was transpiring.

In this keen attentiveness and alertness, I stumbled upon a strange and synchronised movement, starting with the *Ajna chakra,* and catching momentum and activating all the main *chakras* till they were resonating in perfect rhythm. The feeling of the movement is reflected in the physical body as these *chakras* correspond to the main physical organs. There was no discomfort of any sort that was felt. I was being introduced to the *chakras* and their function. I found that when there is a block in the path of the *Kundalini,* it activates the nearby *chakra* and, by increasing its (*chakra's)* speed and pattern of movement suited to the density of the block, it creates an energy which breaks down the block. Clear demonstration of this was given to me when the block in my spleen was completely shattered. I started to learn the *chakra* language, I became sensitive to their change of shape, movement, and rhythm, depending on what the moment demanded. I realised that the blood circulates in the physiological body, nurturing it, whereas *Kundalini* circulates in the etheric body, nurturing the nervous system, and the quality of its circulation and flow affects the physical body.

As I progressed on my spiritual journey, I was constantly warned not to voice my experiences to others because then my progress would stop. I was also told not to dwell on them. My reasoning was that if I was being given a certain experience, it was for a purpose and so for sharing, and if I did not dwell on it, how was I to understand what was being conveyed? "The riddle of the universe is about me and I am now solving it." I could only solve it by going over it again and again and realising the purpose of it. And, also, because the journey was so simple, adventurous, and exhilarating, the need was there for other aspirants to experience the joy of it and add another dimension to their lives.

I also realise now why one is advised to keep the knowledge to oneself. It is mainly to avoid any feeling of self aggrandisement and to prevent undeveloped psyches from experimenting.

My awakening happened through following the course of *Brahma Vidya*. It is a course of study and practice that leads the student towards a meaningful and conscious existence. It helps to de-condition the conditioned mind and, in a few aspirants who are ready, the awakening of *Kundalini* takes place. *Kundalini yoga* is a powerful form of *yoga* and should be undertaken under the guidance of a *Guru* who has travelled the same path.

What I now realise is that during the period of my spiritual unfoldment – I was living simultaneously in the dense physical dimension as well as at the subtle dimension i.e. my *Ida* and *Pingala* and the left and right cortical regions of the brain were working simultaneously. That is how I was able to function at the two dimensions at one and the same time.

"In ordinary life this does not happen because the simultaneous awakening and functioning of life force and consciousness can take place only if the central canal, sushumna, is connected with kundalini, the source of energy. If sushumna can be connected in the physical body, it can reactivate the brain cells and create a new physical structure."

– Saraswati – 'Kundalini Tantra', op. cit., p. 27.

A clear understanding has emerged as to what the words 'awakening' and 'self-realisation' mean. 'Awakening' is to understand the difference between 'conscious' and 'unconscious' living. Awakening means to realise the power of thought and to know that I am the Creator of my destiny. When an individual can cultivate the habit of being always 'in the moment', he is cultivating the practice of living consciously.

The best advice to any serious aspirant who is on the path of self-discovery was by Swami Vivekananda.

"It is wrong to believe blindly. You must exercise your own reason and judgment; you must practise, and see whether these things happen or not... There is neither mystery nor danger in it. So far as it is true, it ought to be preached in the public streets in broad daylight. Any attempt to mystify these things is productive of great danger."

– Vivekananda, Swami – 'Raja Yoga'. Advaita Ashrama, Calcutta, India, 1923. Twenty seventh Impression, 2001, p. 15.

Kundalini awakening should either happen naturally or then under the guidance of a *Guru*. I feel that even if it happens naturally, one needs constant supervision and reassurance from the *Guru* in order to progress. This is so, because during the practices one may enter the realm of the unconscious and experience the inexplicable, hear sounds or see demons. Therefore, the Masters advise that:

"...before you attempt kundalini awakening you should undergo a process of thought purification and develop understanding of your way of thinking."

– Saraswati – 'Kundalini Tantra', op. cit., p. 68.

When the *Kundalini* awakens, there are some simple guidelines one can follow, that will help one map one's progress. They are:

- Not to ignore your experience, as is often advised, because nothing is a figment of imagination.
- Everything that happens has a reason and a purpose. Until you look at it and understand it, you are going to be faced with it again and again, no matter how trivial.
- To become a keen observer of what transpires during your *sadhana.*
- To make note of your experience in a diary.
- To ponder over your notes.
- There is nothing that is irrelevant that you experience during your meditation. Everything has a meaning, an association, and a purpose.
- Everything is emerging from the deepest regions of your memory.
- You are looking into your history and have to be thankful to it for being where you are today.
- As long as your intention is clear, what is unfolding is your route of evolution.
- You can actually map your existence.
- Be without fear.
- Have a definite purpose.
- Exercise surrender.

Once you have completed tracing your life happenings and actualised your desire for which the awakening happened, and there is nothing left for the memory bank to throw up, then the experience or visualising will stop. Only then will there be no outward expression; there will be no more demons, no elephants or serpents, or any other manifestation or *mudras.* There is only the 'isness' of it, because beyond the mind there is only wholeness that cannot be divided. There, the experience, the experiencer, and the experienced do not exist.

...Bring me my horse – my horse? my wings
That I may soar the sky,...
Far as the Future vaults her skies,
From this my vantage ground
To those still-working energies
I spy nor term nor bound.

As we surpass our father's skill,
Our sons will shame our own;
A thousand things are hidden still
And not a hundred known.

And had some prophet spoken true
Of all we shall achieve,
The wonders were so wildly new,
That no man would believe.

Meanwhile, my brothers, work, and wield
The forces of to-day,
And Plough the present like a field,
And garner all you may!

You, what the cultured surface grows,
Dispense with careful hands:
Deep under deep forever goes,
Heaven over heaven expands.

Mechanophilus
– Alfred Lord Tennyson

AFTERWORD

I had been having a series of dialogues with Santosh on my visits to Mumbai since the publication of her first book, *Conscious Flight Into The Empyrean*. Little did I know that a spur-of-the-moment intuition to call her during one of my visits to Mumbai would develop into a deep trusting friendship and exchange of ideas and experiences. Even though I was born and raised in India, my career and life path led me out of India and into several other continents. My spiritual interests led me to explore spiritual traditions from many cultures. I found many beautiful traditions outside of the rich Hindu tradition, such as Tibetan Buddhism, Egyptian Mysteries, Christianity, Western Esotericism, and Native North American teachings, but somehow kept searching for just a little more. At last, I finally found one tradition that allowed me to combine all of my experiences and insights into one approach. Peruvian Shamanism allowed me to take all that I learned, and incorporate it into my *Mesa,* or altar. There are a few requirements for creating the *Mesa,* which are traditionally accepted, but after that, the individual is responsible for building everything else around that core.

For Santosh, her spiritual journey really started by simply asking to know her Source. In the Shamanic tradition, intention is critical. It determines your course and your goal. Energy follows the focus of the mind. It is like focusing the light of the Sun through a magnifying glass to amplify its power to heat. This is excellently exemplified in one of her visions where people are doing circumambulation around her as if she's an idol in a temple. She had so focused her attention that she became the 'Source'.

The purpose of the highest degree of initiation in the Shamanic or mystical path is to understand our oneness with all of life. That is the highest truth we can experience. Above the portal of the temple at Delphi, Greece, was the inscription, "Know Thyself." Many ancient temples had similar instructions. Easy to say or read, but how is this actually accomplished? Fortunately, **Santosh's book outlines her path: serious inquiry, focused attention, meditation, pranayam, contemplation, perseverance, realisation.** Realisation is not a mental understanding but an experience of true inner 'knowing'. When you 'know' anything, there is absolutely no doubt about what you 'know'. When Christ said, "I and my Father are One," it wasn't a wish or prayer. It was a statement of his experience. Further, he claimed no uniqueness for this achievement, but said it was the birthright of all of us, there only for the claiming. When you become one with that which you venerate, you are It!

In the tradition of Peruvian Shamanism that I have been initiated into, you are one with Nature and all its elements. In her 16th October, 1996 meditation, Santosh is in the realm of flowers with different colours and fragrances, and she finds a *Shivalinga* with a golden snake around it. The snake and *Linga* become golden light on the rippling surface of the water. In my own mystical experience of light and energy, when I became one with the essence of all things, I joined in the stream of Light, which I call the "Liquid Universe" as it seems like water by the quality of the energy flowing. The snake and *Linga* are not unique to *Kundalini Tantra* as some may believe. The snake or dragon appear in all mystical traditions and cultures. The *Linga* is also called the Omphalos (navel of the world) stone in ancient traditions of Greece, with similar concepts in Egypt and Mesopotamia. These traditions also display this Omphalos with a snake wrapped around it.

In one of her experiences, Santosh sees a stray unclean dog, which turns into a *Rishi,* who then turns into a starved-looking, bent, bearded *Sadhu*. In the stream of Light of consciousness, when one is One with all things (dog, *Rishi, Sadhu*), one is free to dance and experience the Freedom of Spirit that all inwardly seek. There is *lila,* yet no *lila*. All is Freedom. The opening of a door, in the Shamanic tradition, is a symbol for an opportunity. In the case of one of Santosh's experiences, the opportunity is to leave the ego behind and start what is known as the Shamanic Journey. Ego can't participate in this journey since it prevents the possibility of the journey. The part of us that is needed for this journey is the consciousness of the oneness with all life. The Shaman is the one who can see this unity in all things and help others through being able to function in this "alternate" reality. In the journey, the Shaman becomes the bird or flies with the bird into the *Hanaq Pacha* (Upper World), *Kay Pacha* (Middle World) or *Uju Pacha* (Inner World).

Santosh's experience of wings around her head represents an Upper World experience, following which she experiences an expansion of consciousness and feelings of freedom. Santosh also experiences being stretched into two vibratory levels. This is like being in the Upper (Higher) and Inner (Lower or Subconscious) Worlds, which each person experiences in his or her Shamanic journey towards wholeness. Joseph Campbell described it as the Hero's Journey. First comes the quest (intention), followed by going out (attention/meditation), slaying of dragons (victory over our illusions of separation) and return home (to wholeness). At an inner level, all spiritual seekers take this journey, and for each of us there are inner demons to be slain before truly coming home. Santosh has a profound experience of 'I am This' and 'I am That'. I am stillness and I am also movement. This is directly comparable to the Buddhist concepts of Emptiness (stillness) and Form (movement). There is form or the potential of form in Emptiness or the Great Void or stillness.

Santosh describes the activation of the *Spleen chakra* and the expansion of her etheric body. The spleen is the area where we hold our deep feelings. When we let go of old feelings and habit patterns that no longer serve us, we can become free of the Wheel of *Maya,* or the illusion of separation. That is why she was able to take off as a Spirit of Freedom rising up into space, and become a whole circle swirling and submerging in the Cosmos. When you disperse and become consciousness of the rest of the world, you realise the delight the Creator has in His/Her Creation.

Santosh also experiences becoming one with the elements, Water and Earth. In Shamanic terms, only after you have reconciled your physical (earth), emotional (water) and mental (fire – see 17th May, 1997 experience) components, are you truly prepared to move to the spiritual, or realm of God/Self. This is what she experienced on 18th March, 1997 (pg. 69) as merging of Self with *Guru*/God. Whether one calls it past life *sadhana* or this life purification by fire (i.e. mind), then one is ready, in Shamanic terms, to be one with the *Quichi,* or centre of the Universe (God/Self). Santosh becomes one with Earth energy on

22nd May, 1997. It's not only energy of *Muladhar* but also called *Pachamama* or Mother Earth, or Mother Universe, or Divine Feminine.

As Santosh becomes one with the consciousness of all on 7th July, 1997 she observes Sun worship in prehistoric times. All over the world, in all ancient cultures, there were built great Sun Temples. In Peruvian Shamanism, the Sun Temple, Qorikancha, in Cuzco, Peru, was the centre of the Inca Empire and is the centre of the current Shamanic tradition.

Surrendering of the ego, in the Shamanic tradition, is what allows you to experience oneness with all life and that is what happens to Santosh on 23rd July, 1997 when she surrenders, not to the *Guru's* feet, but to the greater Light. This is followed by birds coming to her. Birds, in the Shamanic tradition, always represent the Spirit (*Hanaq Pacha* or Upper World). The specific birds are pigeon and owl. The pigeon represents the return to love and the true Spiritual Home. Owls represent wisdom. After the birds come, her *Guru* gives her a stone and tells her to keep it on her body. Stones represent *Pachamama* (Mother Earth and the Creative Principle). This is truly a marriage of Heaven (winged ones) and Earth (stone).

On the Peruvian *Mesa* (altar), this would be symbolised by the North (Heaven/Spirit) meeting with the South (Earth/Physical) in the Centre (*Quichi*) of the *Mesa* (Divine Essence). In one of her experiences, Santosh moves in a labyrinth. Labyrinths have been found in most cultures and date back at least four thousand years. They generally incorporate the circle and the spiral, two of the most basic forms of nature. Typically, the way you go in is the way you come out. It is a metaphor for your spiritual journey. On 21st August, 1997 Santosh doesn't know whether she is in meditation or asleep. She asks if she's in the womb and she's told "Yes, the womb of Mother Creation." Only when we leave the consciousness of unity with the Divine does the illusion of our waking dream begin, that greatest of all illusions, the illusion that we're separate from the Divine. The truly Awakened Ones of the past (Krishna, Buddha, Christ) have tried to remind us of our Divine Nature. Let us thank Santosh for hearing the echoes of those Great Masters and responding with her own beginning of wakefulness. Most of all, let us thank her for sharing her experiences. For when one person begins to Wake Up, all of us are that much closer to waking up ourselves.

– Meera Sharma-Seman

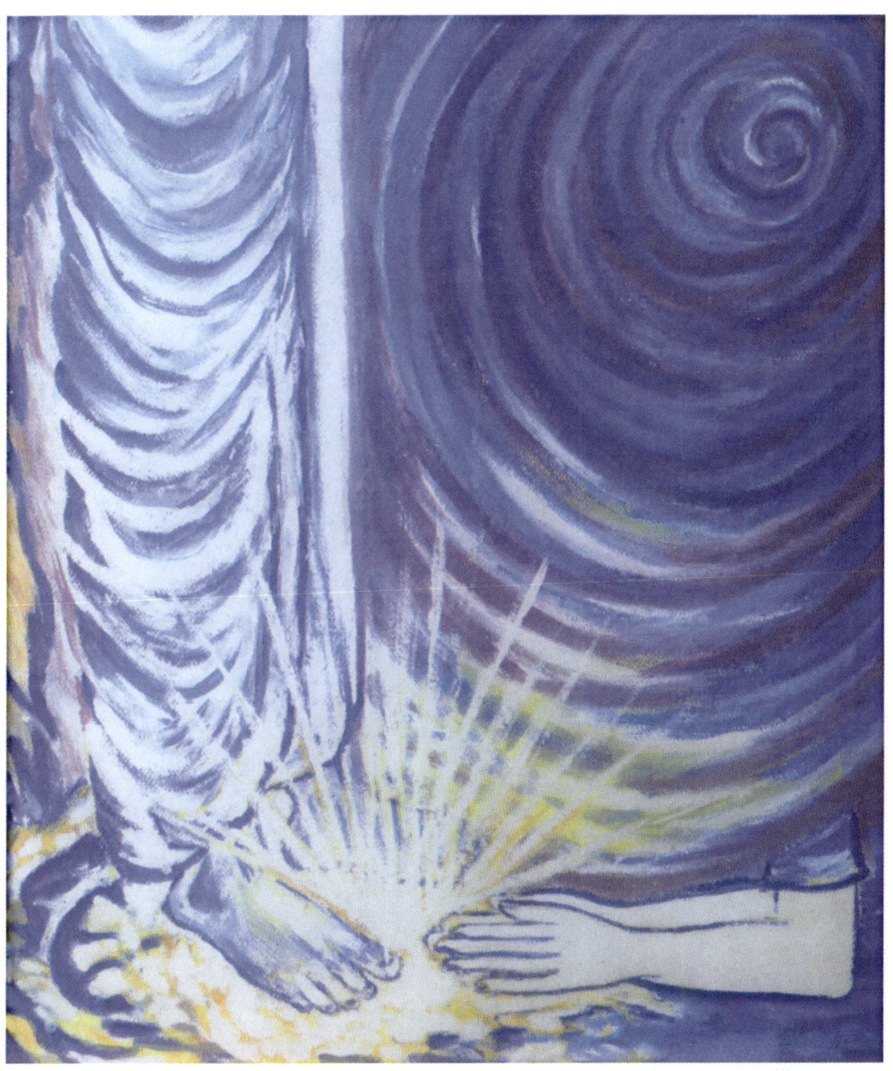

Surrender

THE GURUS

Gurus have been a part of my life from early childhood and through the years, as life has moved on. They have kept pace with me, lending their support through various stages of my growth, whether material or spiritual. However, the Masters whom I have experienced more consciously in the last six years are Justice M. L. Dudhat, Eckhart Tolle, Swami Ramanathan and Ramesh Balsekar, and through my daughter Shibani, Sri Sri Ravi Shankar. All convey the message of love and compassion – the difference lies in the way it is conveyed.

Justice M. L. Dudhat *Guruji* follows the long tradition of householder *Gurus*, people who have gracefully donned the mantle of spiritual service while shouldering the responsibilities of a family and occupation. He was appointed as Judge of the Bombay High Court in 1989, but continued the teaching of *Brahma Vidya* simultaneously. He brought a rare sense of humility and compassion to his role as a judge, even embracing, with deep sensitivity, the convicts summoned to his chambers, against whom he had passed the death sentence just a short while earlier. His genuine ability as a true Master is reflected in his sense of detachment and equipoise.

With love, tenderness, patience, and a non-judgemental attitude, he enabled the creativity within me to surface, and awakened feelings of love and surrender. He is, and has been, a very real nurturing, accepting, and reassuring presence in my own life as well as the lives of my children.

Master Charles was fully instructed in the eastern mystical tradition in India by *Paramahamsa* Muktananda. As genuine mystical illumination continued to unfold in his Master's energy field, he recognised his destiny as a bridge across two very different cultures – bringing home to the West the experiential understanding that freedom, peace, and bliss are our true nature and the birthright of every human being. Master Charles is recognised worldwide as the originator of a contemporary context of meditation, the Synchronicity High-Tech Meditation Experience. Master Charles tackles the ego with great clarity of word and thought. He does not spare your sentiments or your sensitivities. His approach is a 'no nonsense' approach, and his energy field is electric. He will not allow you to hide behind any fabricated illusions.

My association with him is through my daughter Nikki. Before going into publishing the books about my experiences, I went to different Masters seeking clarification about whether they should be published. I did not get any answers. When I wrote to Master Charles, he wrote back: *"In the tradition of enlightening Masters, it is said that one should not reveal their experiences until they have the command of their master to do so. These Masters are just calling your attention to this protocol to ensure that you are clear within yourself that the sharing of your experience be from the highest dimensions of your Sourceful self and not merely from any egotistical expression. It seems to me that your intention is Sourceful and therefore your book has come into manifestation as a direct result. This is indeed appropriate. Therefore, I am sure it will assist many and your ongoing journey of ever enlightening awareness will continue."*

I remain ever grateful to Master Charles for lending clarity to my confusion.

Ramesh Balsekar talks on the Advaita philosophy. The concept he puts forth is, "All there is, is Consciousness." In that original state – call it Reality, call it Absolute, call it Nothingness – there was no reason to be aware of anything. So, Consciousness-at-rest was not aware of itself. It became aware of itself only when this sudden feeling, 'I Am' arose. 'I Am' is the impersonal sense of being aware. And that was when Consciousness-at-rest became Consciousness-in-movement, when potential energy became actual energy. They are not two. Nothing separate comes out of the potential energy.

Eckhart Tolle is the author of the powerful book, *The Power of Now*. Eckhart has the gentlest, softest, most powerful and extensive energy field. In his embrace, I felt like a miniscule particle in the vast ocean of love. For me two lines from his book sum up his teachings:

"Nothing ever happened in the past; it happened in the Now.
Nothing will ever happen in the future; it will happen in the Now."

– Tolle, Eckhart – 'The Power of Now'. Yogi Impressions Books Pvt. Ltd., Mumbai, India. First India printing, 2001, p. 41.

Guru Jyotirmayananda (Swami Ramanathan) is the founder of the Brahma Vidya Mission in India. Being with him is an experience in itself. His body is so energised that his hair stands on end. He uses this vast reservoir of energy for healing. He is love personified in action and word.

On one of my visits I asked him, "Baba, I have heard that when an aspirant reaches a certain stage in his *sadhana,* there are certain secrets that are revealed to him. What are those secrets?"

Baba's answer was, "What you did not know before and is revealed to you now – is the secret."

Param Pujya Swami Gagangirinath Maharaj, on going through the book of my experiences, remarked: "This is a rarest of rare occurances, a *mahadurlabh yoga* in the physical world. The reason for her being singled out for this honour is that she too has been a part of the stream of *Sadhus,* life after life, and this is the culmination of her own *punyakarma* involving hundreds of years of *sadhana.* Every single atom of her body has become receptive to the teachings of the Masters, and this book is the result." It was in his energy field that I felt that my whole personality went through a shift, like a puzzle being dismantled and rearranged. The Breath was given a direction, which led to further unfoldment of knowledge. Baba gave me his blessings. Being in his presence is to experience life at its most bubbling self.

PHOTO ALBUM

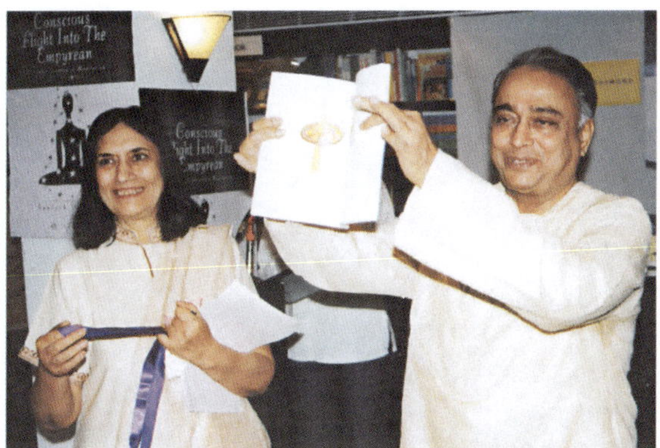

With my Guru at the launch of 'Conscious Flight Into The Empyrean', in 2000.

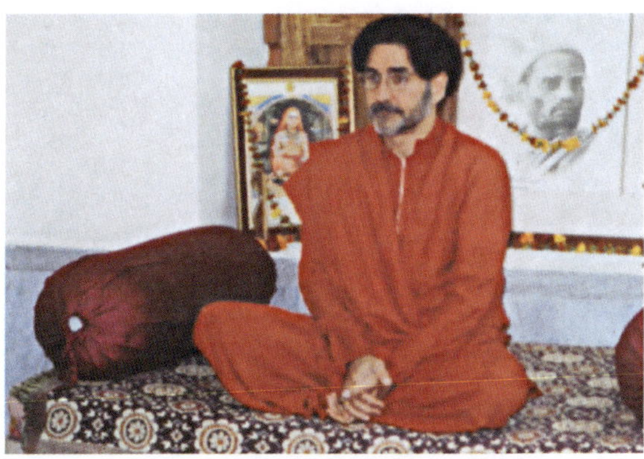

Master Charles at an ashram in North India, in 1998.

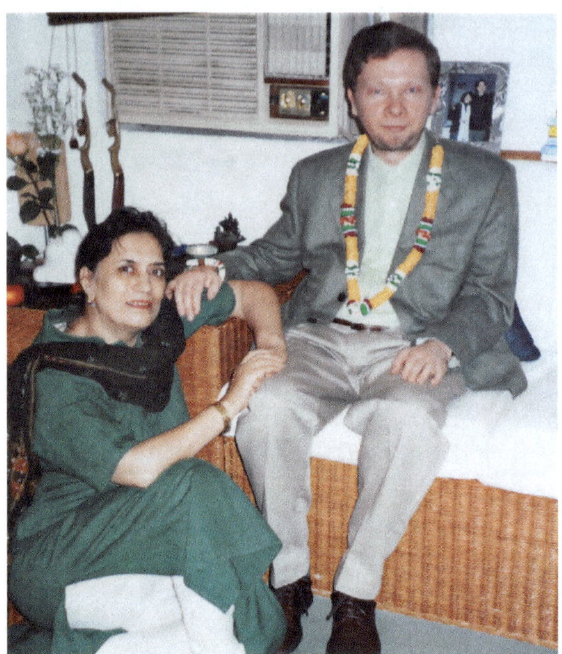

With Eckhart Tolle, at my daughter's home in Hong Kong, November 2000.

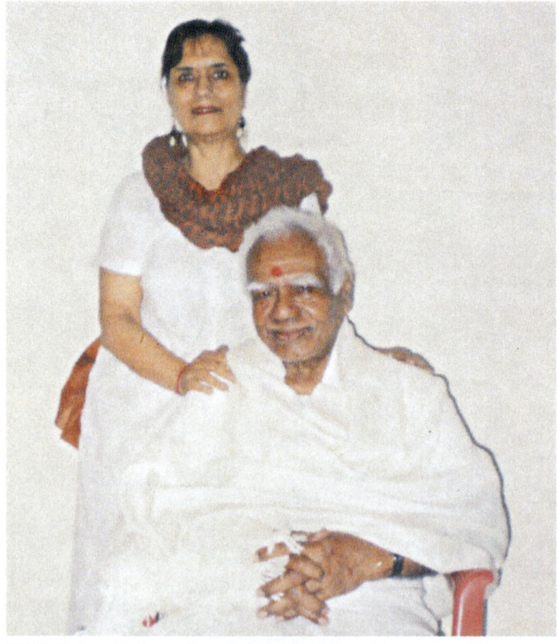

With beloved Guru Jyotirmayananda at his home, July 2001.

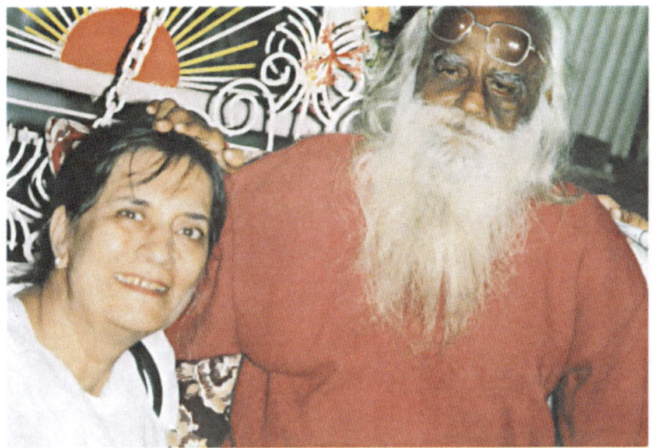

Seeking the blessings of Baba Gagangiri, in 1999.

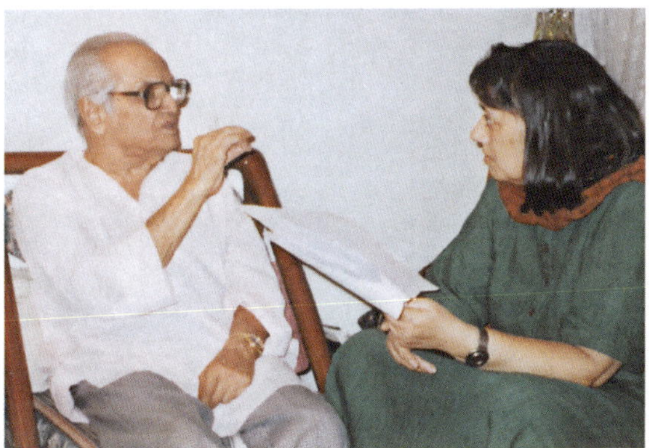

In conversation with Ramesh Balsekar at my home, discussing notes for the second volume, 'Kundalini Diary', in 2000.

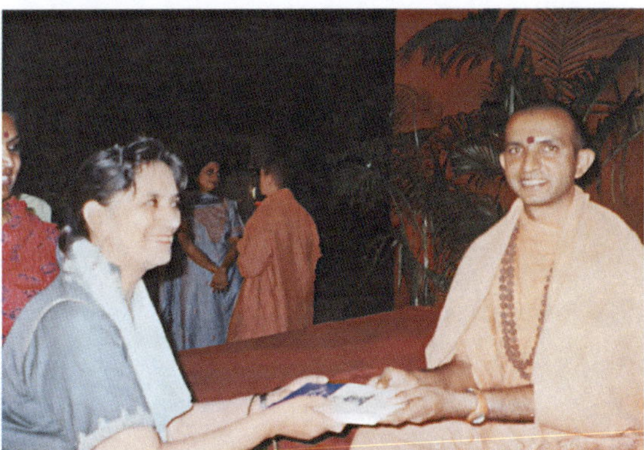

Presenting a copy of my first book to Paramahamsa Swami Niranjanananda Saraswati, President – Bihar School of Yoga, in 2003.

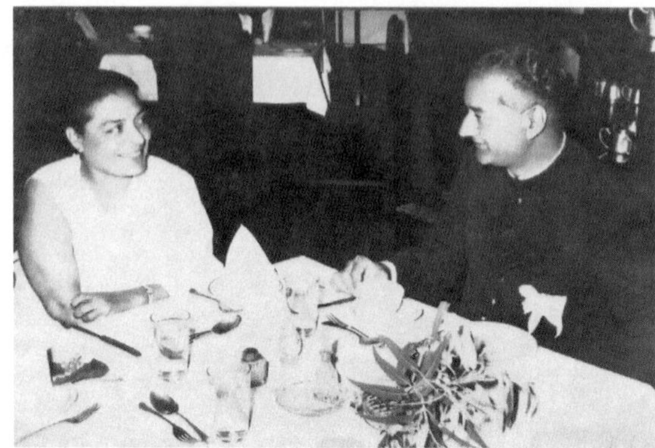

My parents – Janki Devi and Om Prakash Sharma, in 1960.

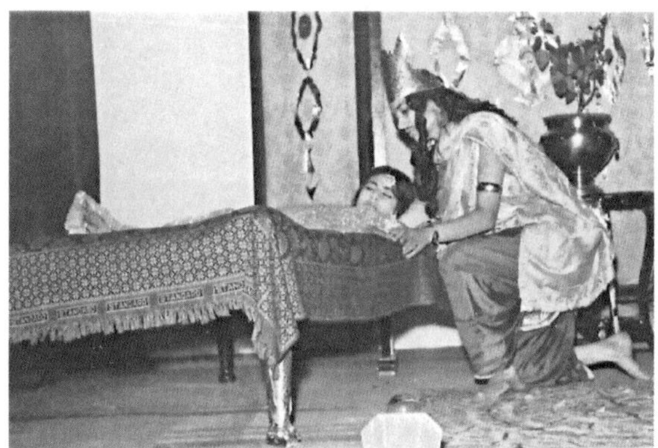

Scene from 'Gautam Buddha' – Staged in 1964. Siddhartha bidding farewell to his wife and new-born son. I played the part of Siddhartha.

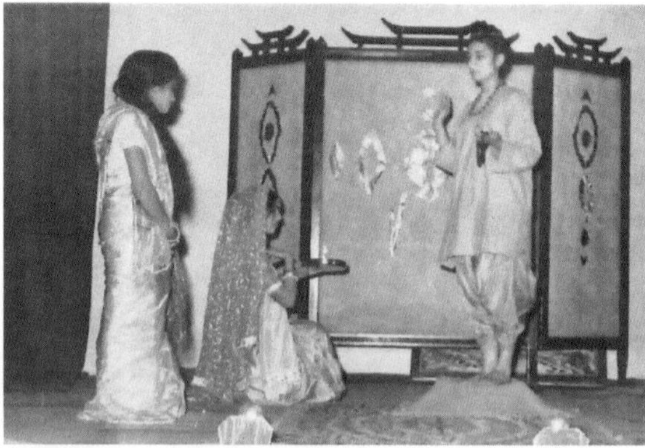

The final scene – Gautam Buddha visits his wife after attaining 'nirvana'.

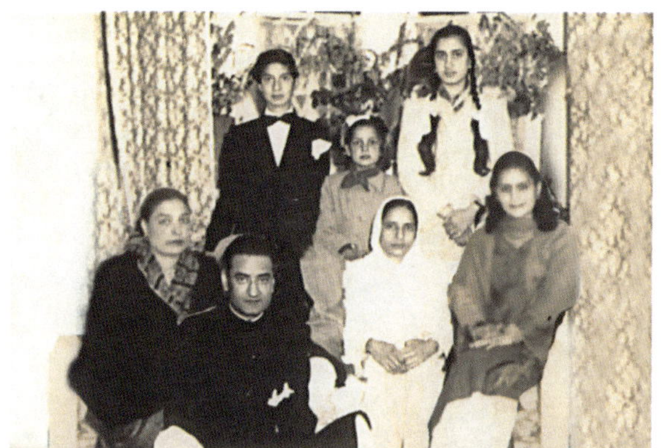

Family photograph at the Savoy Hotel, Mussoorie, 1958.

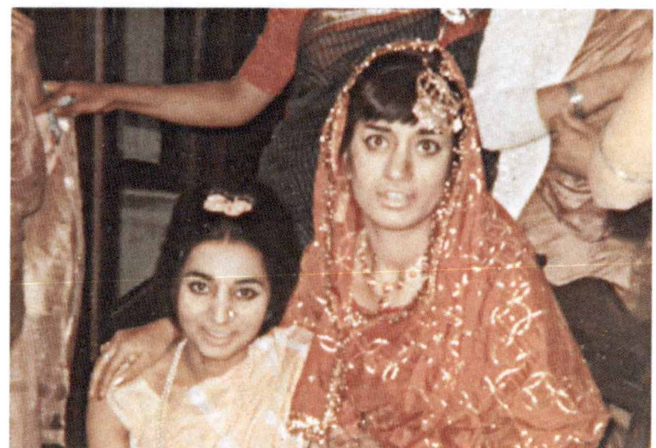

On my wedding day, with my friend Opi, April 1966.

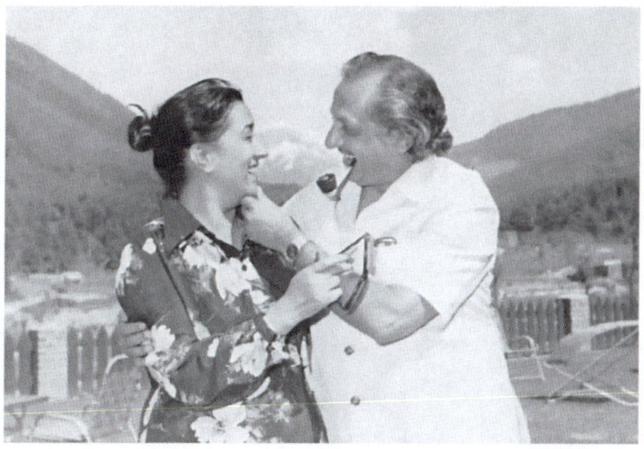

My husband Ajeet and I on holiday in Pahalgam, Kashmir, in 1980.

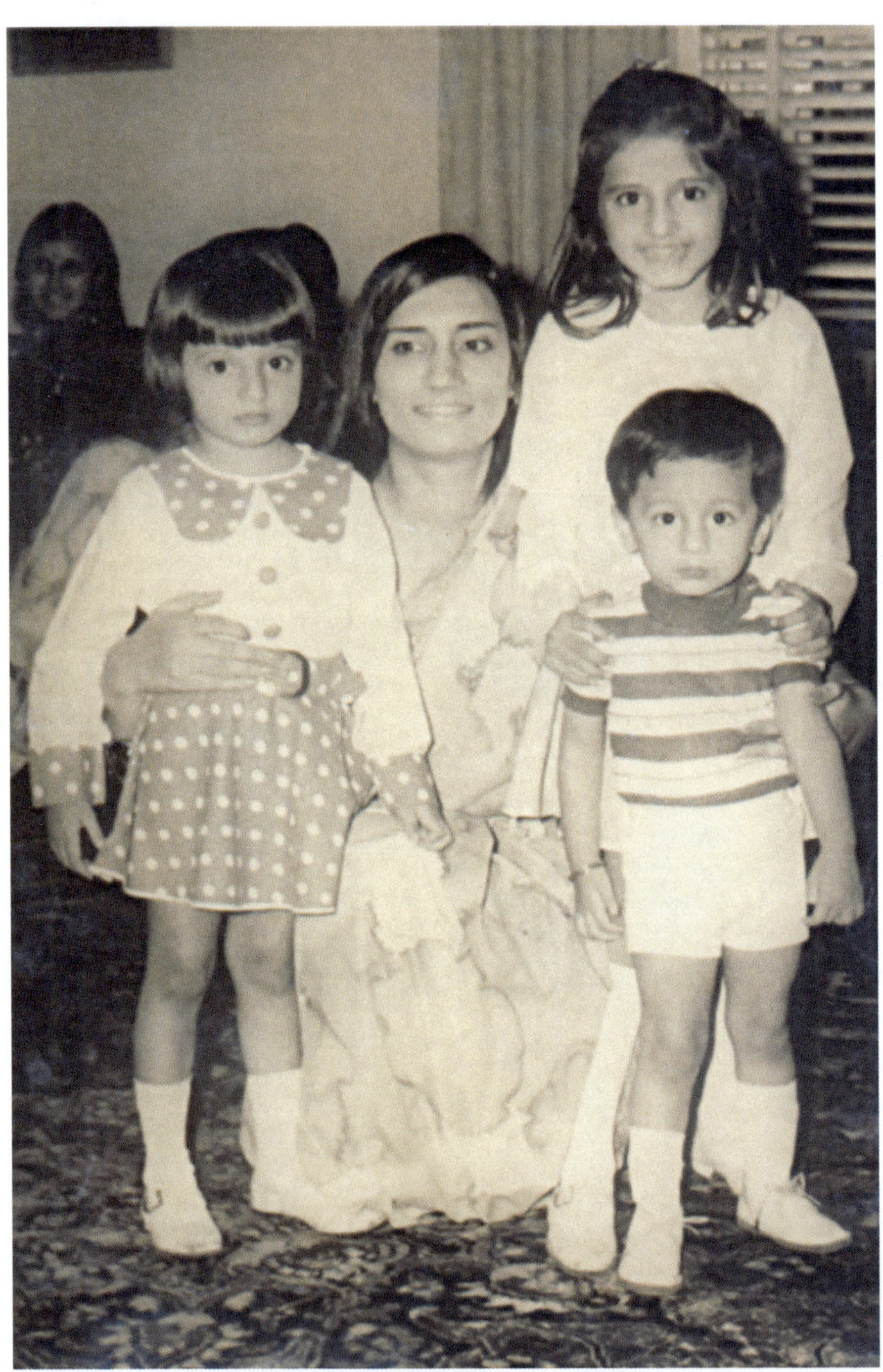

With my children Shibani, Nikki, and Gautam, in 1974.

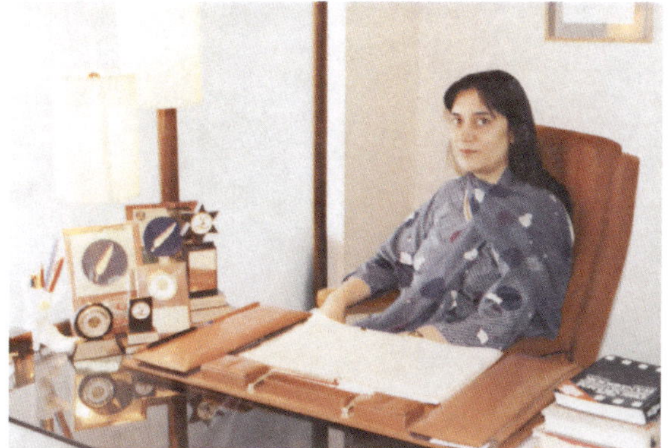

At my office desk, in 1988.

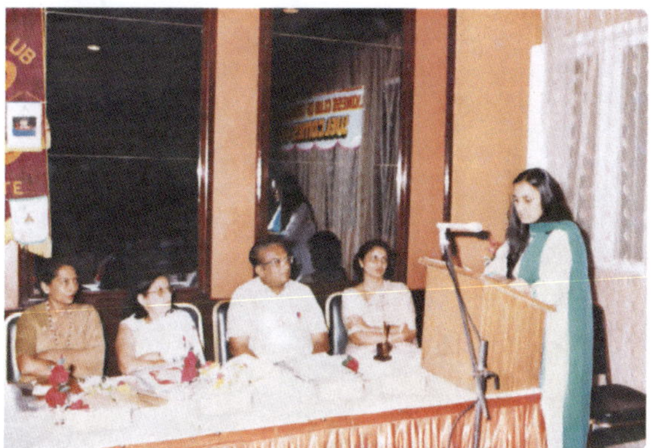

Addressing a meeting as Secretary of The Lioness Club of Churchgate.

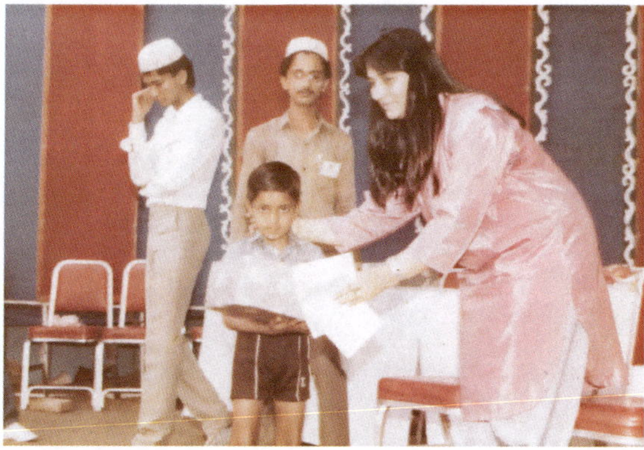

As the chief guest, I hand out a prize to a student at a function organised by the Mandasaur Savings & Credit Society, Byculla.

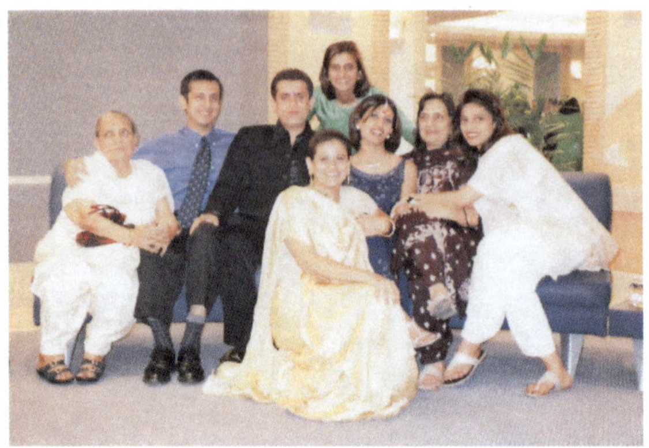

Our family portrait at the engagement of my nephew Vishal, in 2001.

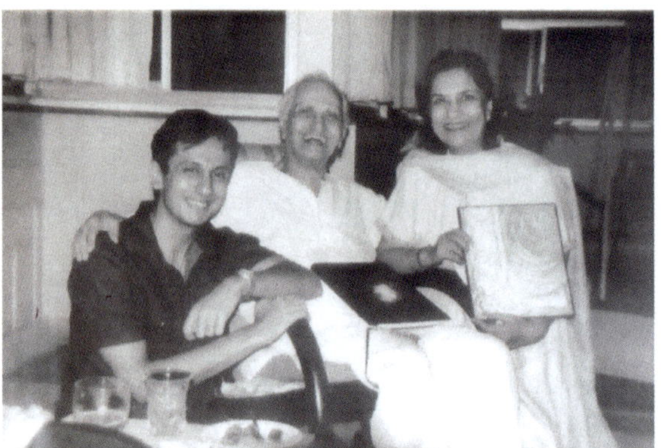

Gautam and I with Ramesh Balsekar at his residence in Mumbai, on his birthday, in 2001.

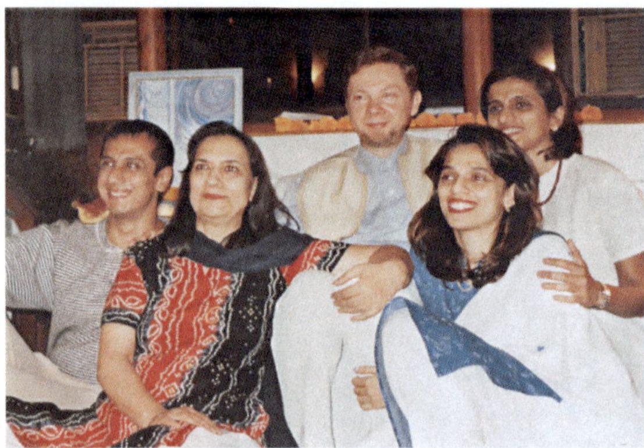

My children and I with Eckhart Tolle at my residence in Mumbai, 2002.

BIBLIOGRAPHY

Ashish – 'The Eternal Culture of the Masters'. Shree Gagangiri Prakashan, Khopoli, India, July 1995.

Balsekar, Ramesh – 'The Whole Truth'. May 1979.

Besant, Annie – 'Man and his Bodies'. The Theosophical Publishing House, Adyar, India, 1896. Second Edition.

Besant, Annie & Leadbeater, C. W. – 'Thought Forms'. The Theosophical Publishing House, Adyar, India, 1925. Tenth Reprint, 1992.

Dunn, Jean – 'Prior to Consciousness – Talks with Sri Nisargadatta Maharaj'. Chetana Pvt. Ltd., Mumbai, India. First Indian Edition, 1998.

Goslin, Robert – Synchronicity Inner Network #714.

Govindan, Marshall – 'Babaji and the 18 Siddha Kriya Yoga Tradition'. Babaji's Kriya Yoga Order of Acharyas Trust, Malleswaram West, Bangalore, India, 2003.

Leadbeater, C. W. – 'A Text Book of Theosophy'. The Theosophical Publishing House, Adyar, India, 1912. Fourteenth Reprint, 1997.

Leadbeater, C. W. – 'Dreams: What they are and how they are caused'. The Theosophical Publishing House, Adyar, India, 1898. Fifteenth Reprint, 1997.

Leadbeater, C. W. – 'Man Visible and Invisible'. The Theosophical Publishing House, Adyar, India, 1925. Eighth Reprint, 1999.

Leadbeater, C. W. – 'The Chakras: A Monograph'. The Theosophical Publishing House, Adyar, India, 1927. Thirteenth Reprint, 1996.

Mookerjee, Ajit – 'Kundalini: The Arousal of the Inner Energy'. Thames and Hudson Ltd., London, 1982. Reprinted, 1995.

Muktibodhananda, Swami – 'Hatha Yoga Pradipika'. Yoga Publication Trust, Munger, Bihar, India, 1985. Reprinted, 2000.

Nityanand, Swami – 'Symbolism in Hinduism'. Central Chinmaya Mission Trust, Mumbai, India, 1983. Third Edition, 1993.

'Osho Zen Tarot – The Transcendental Game of Zen'. St. Martin's Press, 175 Fifth Avenue, New York, 1994. Second Edition.

Patel, Dadubhai N. – 'The Real Essence of Tantra'. Yogi Divine Society, Bombay, India, 1978.

Ramanathan, Swami K. S. – 'Mental Physics: Lectures and Lessons'. (Private circulation), Bombay, India, 1980.

Saraswati, Swami Satyananda – 'Kundalini Tantra'. Bihar School of Yoga, Munger, Bihar, India, 1984. Reprinted, 2000.

Saraswati, Swami Satyananda – 'Yoga Nidra'. Bihar School of Yoga, Munger, Bihar, India, 1976. Sixth Edition, 1998.

Sivananda, Swami – 'Concentration and Meditation'. The Divine Life Society, U.P., India. Eighth Edition, 1990.

Svoboda, Robert E. – 'Kundalini Aghora II'. Rupa & Co., Calcutta, India, 1993. Third Impression, 1996.

Tolle, Eckhart – 'The Power of Now'. Yogi Impressions Books Pvt. Ltd., Mumbai, India. First India printing, 2001.

Vivekananda, Swami – 'Raja Yoga'. Advaita Ashrama, Calcutta, India, 1923. Twenty seventh Impression, 2001.

Woodroffe, Sir John – 'The Serpent Power'. Ganesh & Company, Madras, India. First Paperback Edition, 1995.

GLOSSARY

Agni-Snan Literally, 'The Fire Bath', a purification process practiced by *tantriks.*

ahamkara The sense of the egotistic self.

Alakh Niranjan A chant meaning "Unnoticeable, unmarked, invisible, and pure," as traits characterising the Absolute. Actually, the significative chant of the mendicant ascetics of the Navnath sect.

Amrutha Manthan The churning of the ocean, one of the great myths of the Hindus.

asanas *Yogic* postures.

Aum, Om The all-pervading sound of the cosmic vibrations; the origin of all Creation; a symbolic manifestation of the Infinite Reality or God.

Aum Satyam Aum *Mantra* invoking the Truth *(Satyam).*

aura Energy fields that surround the human organism, visible with heightened spiritual consciousness or by the practice of energy-healing work.

Axis Mundi The Axis of the World or the Cosmic Pillar.

Bhakti The path of devotion to achieve God-realisation.

Bhakti yoga The *yoga* of devotion, generally regarded as most suitable for the modern age.

bij mantras "seed mantras" or sounds which have no particular meaning but have been observed by *yogis* to produce certain powerful results upon chanting. For example, ***"Hrim Shrim."***

bindi Dot or decorative mark worn on the forehead by Hindu women.

Brahma The Creator-God of Hinduism. One of the Hindu Trinity.

Brahma Vidya Knowledge of the Self.

chaakki Grinding stone.

chakra Wheel or disc; in *yogic* literature, one of the several centres of consciousness located in the etheric body, usually depicted as a lotus flower.

chitta Mind; conscious, subconscious and unconscious levels of the brain.

churidar-pyjama Traditional dress worn by Indian men and women.

Dattatreya A composite aspect of God, incorporating the forms of *Shiva, Vishnu,* and *Brahma.*

Devanagri The script in which Sanskrit and Hindi are written.

devas Gods; ethereal beings inhabiting the *devalok.*

dhoti Traditional dress for men worn from the waist downward, made from cotton or silk.

Durga Fierce Warrior-Goddess regarded as the supreme power in the universe by some sects of Hinduism.

Ganpati *Ganesha,* the elephant-headed God of knowledge, arts, wisdom, and auspiciousness, who removes obstacles and prospers all undertakings. Hence, it is mandatory to pray to him when beginning all new ventures.

granthi The three psychic knots on the *sushumna nadi* which hinder the upward passage of *Kundalini – Brahma granthi, Vishnu granthi,* and *Rudra granthi.*

Guru Teacher or guide, who removes the darkness of ignorance, bringing realisation to the disciple.

Guruji Respectful term of address for one's *Guru.*

Hall of the Akashik Records Hall of memories; a supernatural location in the subtle dimensions of the universe where, purportedly, each human life is recorded in excruciating detail. The Individual Consciousness visits it in the after-life to scrutinise and review its *karmic* record and avoid similar mistakes in future incarnations.

Hanuman *Vaanara* God of strength and wisdom, chief devotee of *Ram.*

Hiranyagarbha The 'Golden Egg' principle of all creation, and a great cultural motif in the texts of ancient India.

Ida One of the two main channels (lunar and left) within the body through which the *Kundalini* ascends.

Jyotirlinga *Lingas* formed of light.

Kali Ancient Black Goddess of war beloved of the *tantriks* and regarded as personifying the Absolute by many sects. Her worship seems somewhat bizarre, but all actions are overlaid with symbolic meanings accessible only to those in the know.

karma Based on the principle of reincarnation, the system of Divine Justice whereby people face the results of their positive and negative thoughts and actions.

karmic Pertaining to *karma* and its unfolding.

Krishna *Avatar* of *Vishnu* and his most popular form in terms of worship.

Kriya yoga An extremely effective form of *yoga* popularised by the great *Swami* Yogananda. It emphasises breathing exercises, *yogic* postures, and meditation upon *Vedantic* principles.

Kubera The Hindu God of wealth.

kumkum Red powder applied to the forehead by worshippers, and also used to denote marital status in women.

Kundalini Manifestation of the dynamic female cosmic energy within the individual body, lying nascent in a coiled form at the base of the spine.

Kundalini Tantra Systems or texts dedicated to the *Kundalini.*

Kundalini yoga A branch of *yoga* which is inner directed and is concerned primarily with the awakening of the *Kundalini* and its consequent spiritual experiences.

kurta The typical Indian shirt.

Laxmi Hindu Goddess of prosperity and wife of *Vishnu.*

lila Literally 'play'. Actions performed by God in joy.

linga The symbolic form in which Shiva is worshipped; see *Shivalinga.*

mahadurlabh Extremely difficult to attain.

Maha Tattva The Great Elements, i.e. Earth, Water, Fire, Air, and Ether.

manas buddhi The mind of man or Human Intelligence.

Maya Powers of illusion and creativity associated with *Vishnu;* a veil that prevents the realisation of spiritual truth.

Meru Danda The Cosmic Axis represented in the human body as the spinal column.

Mudras Positions of fingers relative to the palm, common to both *yoga* and classical dance, each *mudra* having a unique symbolic meaning.

nada Sound, usually implying a haunting resonance. Also used as a synonym for the universe which is supposed to be composed of sound.

nadi Etheric channel for energy flow within the body. Out of a total of 35 million *nadis* in a human body, there are 100 major ones. Among these, there are three main *nadis:* the *pingala* or the solar *nadi,* on the right side of the spinal column; the *ida* or the lunar *nadi,* located on the left side; and the most important one of all, the central *nadi,* called the *sushumna,* the vehicle of balanced energy flow, indicative of spiritual growth.

Navratri A festival of nine nights, primarily dedicated to Goddess *Durga* and *Sri Ram.*

Omkara The sacred sound of *Om.*

Padma Lotus; another name for *Laxmi;* a posture in *yoga.*

pandit Learned *Brahmin* who has mastered many of the sacred texts.

Paramahamsa The Supreme Swan. The swan is a bird, venerated in Hindu mythology, for its powers of discrimination; thus the title *Paramahamsa* indicates impeccable spiritual lineage of one who has the ability to discriminate between the Absolute Reality and the illusory world of *maya.*

Pingala One of the two main channels (solar and right) within the body through which the *Kundalini* ascends.

pradakshina Circumambulation of the shrine in a temple.

Prana Life Force or vital energy, which constitutes the breath in living beings.

pranayama The breath control exercises of *yoga* to gain mastery over the *Prana*.

Pranic Pertaining to *Prana*.

puja thali A flat plate upon which is arranged the items for ritual worship.

punyakarma Good deeds accruing over several lifetimes of a person as positive *karma*, bringing into operation the aspect of divine Grace.

rajas The quality and character type of activity and energy.

rishi A sage who has realised the *Brahman*. There are distinctions of expertise amongst *rishis*.

sadhana Adoption of meditation, asceticism, and devotional practices on the spiritual path.

Sadhu Holy man; renunciate; wandering mendicant on a pilgrimage.

sadhvis Feminine of *sadhu*.

Samadhi One of the final stages of meditation, when the aspirant enters what appears to be a trance state, usually with an absence of a body or ego consciousness; the experience in meditation of Oneness and Cosmic Unity.

Sardarji Respectful term of address for *Sikh* males, identified by their distinctive turbans and beards.

sat-chit-ananda A ritual term denoting Existence-Consciousness-Absolute Bliss and one of the highest spiritual stages that the enlightened dwell in.

sattva The quality and character type of purity, positivity, and light.

Shaivites The worshippers of *Shiva*.

Shakti Literally 'strength', but used as a synonym for the creative power of the universe which is female, as well as a generic name for any Goddess including the *Kundalini*.

Shirdi Small town associated with Sai Baba, one of the most powerful Masters of the last century.

Shiva One of the Hindu Trinity, the androgynous God of destruction.

Shivalinga Representation of the union of the male and female principles, symbolising Creation. Worshipped in stone, in the phallic form as *Lord Shiva* who Himself is half-female.

siddha A person perfected in *yoga*; a group of semi-legendary *yogic* masters of India with great spiritual accomplishments.

siddhis Powers that arise within the person with the rigorous practice of *yoga*. They are signposts of accomplishment, but also distractions from the ultimate goal of liberation. Clairvoyance and levitation are two of the more interesting *siddhis*.

Sikh A member of a particular religious sect with the distinguishing characteristic of wearing a turban and beard.

Spleen chakra It is not indicated in the traditional texts, but its place is taken by a centre called the *Swadhisthan*, situated in the area of the generative organs.

Sushumna The nadi, or energy channel, that leads to the sacral *chakra*, the *Sushumna.*

Swami Title used to address a God-realised person of one of the several monastic orders who practices renunciation, celibacy, and asceticism, and who represents spiritual authority.

tamas The quality and character type of inertia, darkness, and sloth.

tandav The great dance of *Shiva*.

Tanmatra Physical senses like smell, taste, sight, hearing, and touch.

Tantra A method or system of worship and prayer practiced in India, Nepal, and Tibet.

tantrik One who practices *Tantra;* pertaining to *Tantra.*

Tattva Literally, 'basic stuff', i.e. element.

thanka A Tibetan wall hanging, normally intricately painted.

tika/tilak A mark applied on the forehead to signify one's sectarian status.

tratak Concentrated gaze on a spot.

trishul Trident, a weapon associated with *Shiva.*

tulsi The most sacred plant in the Indian ethos, regarded as an independent deity. Its leaves have medicinal properties.

Vaishnavites The worshippers of *Vishnu.*

Vedas The holiest books of the Hindus, four in number, *Rig Veda, Sama Veda, Yajur Veda* and *Atharva Veda,* circa 2700 BCE – 1500 BCE, regarded as divine and 'seen' by the seers rather than revealed. The *Vedas* are eternal and survive cosmic dissolution.

Vishnu Literally, 'He who pervades'. One of the Hindu Trinity. Famed as the Protector and Rescuer.

Yagna The famous fire sacrifice of the Hindus, regarded as the most auspicious activity possible, and the only infallible method of communicating with the Gods.

yantra An abstract geometric pattern which signifies the unique characteristics of a deity or group of deities.

Yogi Anyone who practices *yoga* as a method of divine realisation, whether he or she is a renunciate or a householder.

Yoni Literally, 'Womb', but represented as an inverted triangle, the perennial symbol of the Great Mother.

Yupa Stambha the sacrificial post at the fire sacrifice, signifying the Cosmic Axis around which the Universe revolves.

For information on Santosh Sachdeva, visit:
www.santoshsachdeva.com

The author may be contacted on email:
mails@santoshsachdeva.com

For further details, contact:
Yogi Impressions LLP
1711, Centre 1, World Trade Centre,
Cuffe Parade, Mumbai 400 005, India.

Fill in the Mailing List form on our website and receive, via email, information on books, authors, events and more.
Visit: www.yogiimpressions.com

Telephone: (022) 40115981, 22155036
E-mail: yogi@yogiimpressions.com

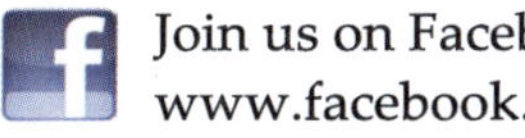

Join us on Facebook:
www.facebook.com/yogiimpressions

Join us on Instagram:
www.instagram.com/yogi_impressions

OTHER TITLES FROM SANTOSH SACHDEVA PUBLISHED BY YOGI IMPRESSIONS

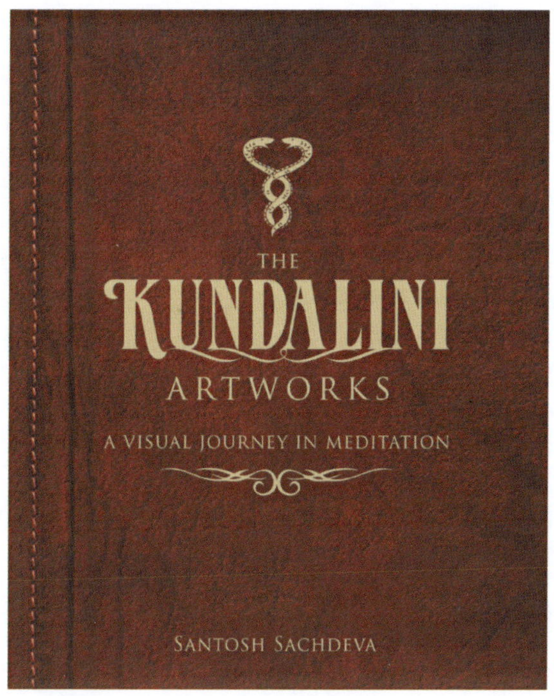

Several readers of the author's earlier three books forming 'The Kundalini Trilogy' observed that just looking at the visuals depicting the visions seen during her meditations had triggered the Kundalini energy that had been lying dormant in them. It was then realised that the visuals themselves took on the role of the Guru (the Kundalini Shakti), enabling aspirants to walk along 'Its' path and progress on their spiritual journey. So it was decided to bring all the illustrations together in *The Kundalini Artworks* in the pristine state as Santosh saw and drew them. To achieve this, the supporting textual entries in 'The Kundalini Trilogy' have been removed. The visuals resonate with a powerful spiritual energy of their own.

Size: 8.5″ × 11″ • Full Colour • Art Paper • Hardbound • Limited Edition

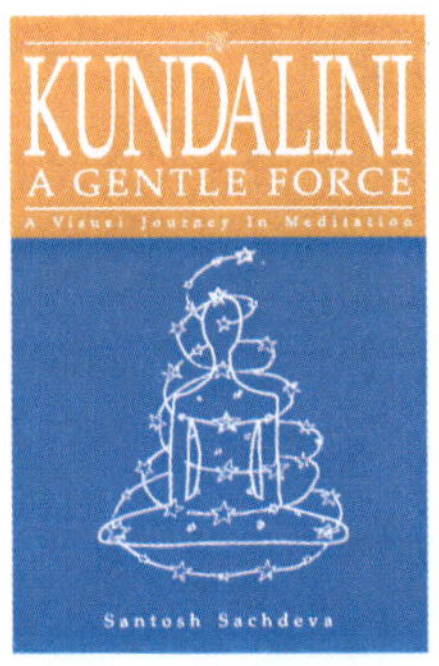

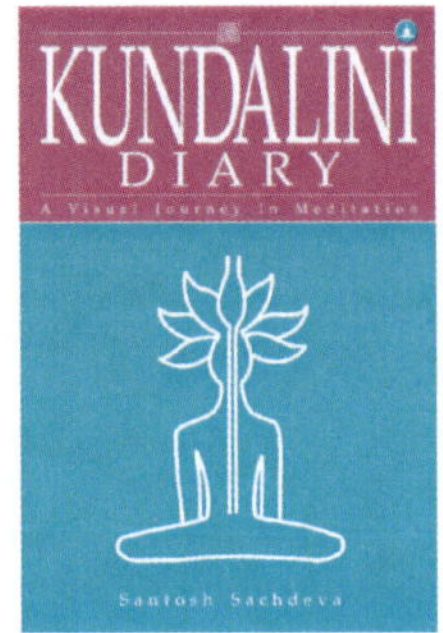

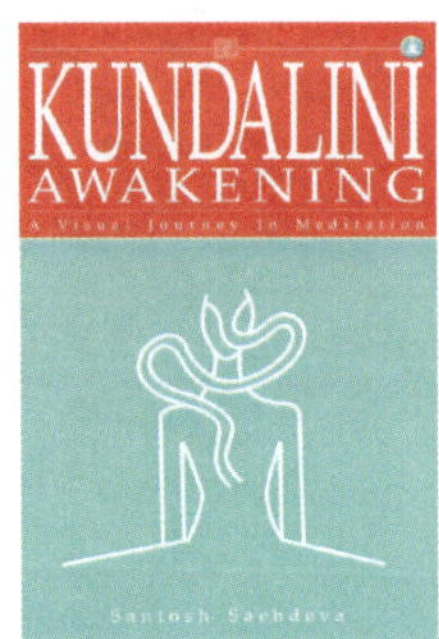

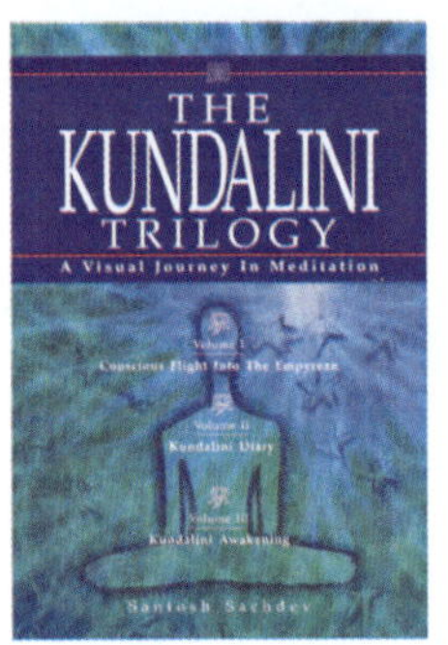

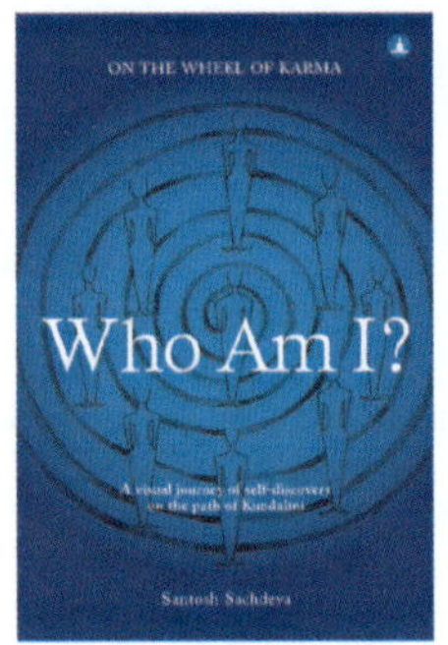

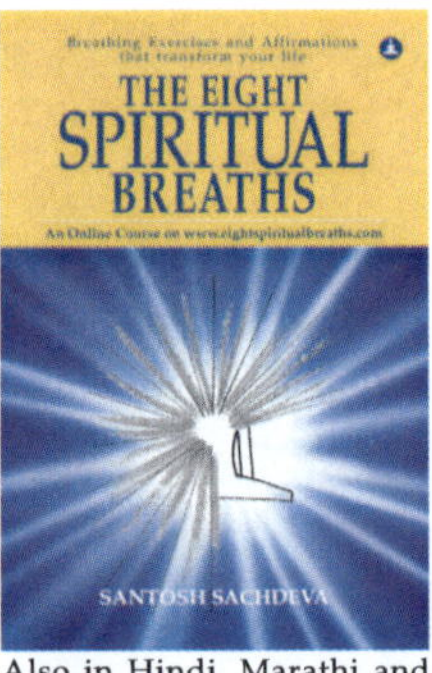

Also in Hindi, Marathi and Gujarati.

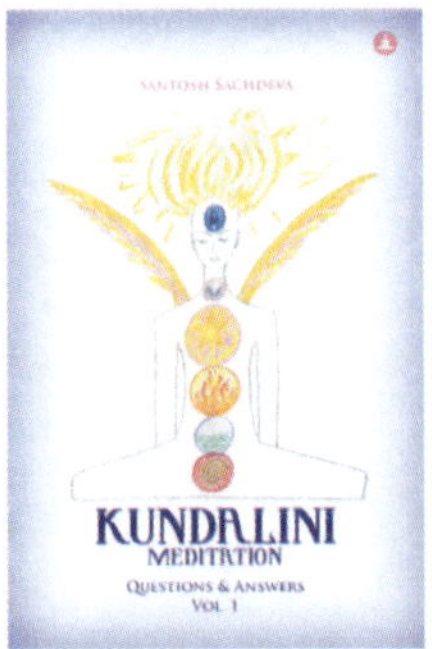

Also in Hindi and Marathi.

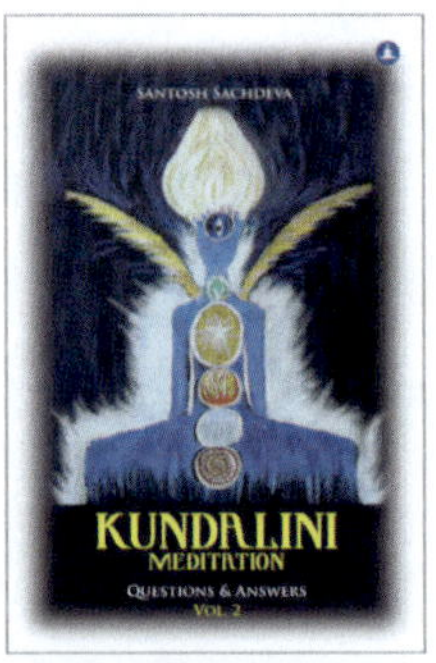

Also in Hindi and Marathi.

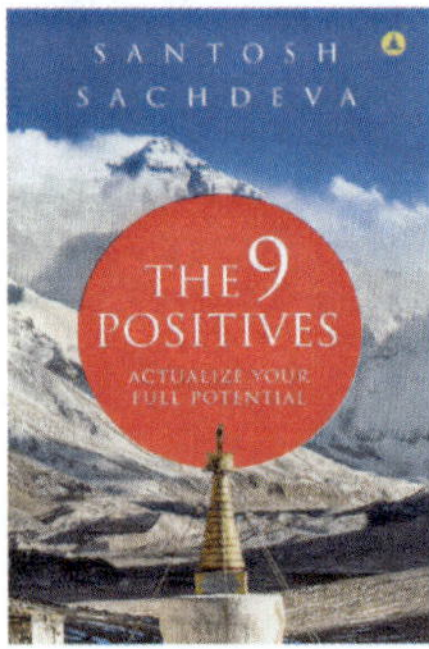

Also in Hindi and Marathi.

THE KUNDALINI PRINTS

These illustrations have been specially chosen by Santosh Sachdeva from *The Kundalini Trilogy* and represent some of the key processes in Kundalini awakening.

Available on www.yogiimpressions.com